GOD's NUTRITIONIST

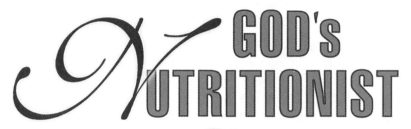

GOD's NUTRITIONIST

Pearls of Wisdom from Ellen G. White

Edited by Robert Cohen

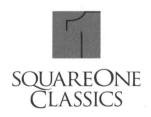

SQUAREONE
CLASSICS

Cover Designer: Phaedra Mastrocola
Typesetter: Gary A. Rosenberg
In-House Editor: Marie Caratozzolo

Square One Publishers
115 Herricks Road
Garden City Park, NY 11040
(516) 535–2010 • (877) 900-BOOK
www.squareonepublishers.com

Library of Congress Cataloging-in-Publication Data

White, Ellen Gould Harmon, 1827–1915.
 God's nutritionist / Ellen G. White ; Robert Cohen, editor.
 p. cm.
 ISBN 0-7570-0146-7 (pbk.)
 1. Vegetarianism—Religious aspects—Christianity. I. Cohen, Robert. II. Title.
BT749.W48   2004
241'.693—dc22

                                        2004004928

Printed in the United States of America

10 9 8 7 6 5 4 3 2 1

Contents

Acknowledgments, ix

Preface, xi

Foreword, xv

Introduction, 1

Quotations, 7

Words to Live By, 168

Concluding Thoughts, 169

Ten Rules for Better Health Care, 171

To my father, Nathan Cohen,
who, at the age of eighty-six,
became a vegetarian;
And to my mother, Dorothy,
whose love evolved eighty years of cooking skills
into the creation of vegetarian art.

Acknowledgments

"If I have seen further than you and Descartes,
it is by standing upon the shoulders of giants."
—Sir Isaac Newton (1675)

I owe a mountain of gratitude to friends, colleagues, and loved ones, whose shoulders are often fatigued by my quenchless desire for a better view.

For teaching me the basics of neurology, physiology, endocrinology, diet, and nutrition: Robert Orndoff, T. Colin Campbell, John McDougall, Glen Merzer, Harvey Diamond, Douglas Graham, Neal Barnard, Hans Diehl, Kim Balas, H. J. Roberts, Michael Greger, Julian Whitaker, George Eisman, Jane Heimlich, Joel Fuhrman, and my Southampton College professors.

For teaching me the basics of cooking: Mom, Ken Bergeron, Ron Pickarski, David Wolfe, Joanne Stepaniak, Brad Wolff, and my instructors at the Culinary Institute of America in Hyde Park, New York.

For teaching me that animals have the ability to feel pain: Kimber Gorall, Howard Lyman, Bruce Friedrich, Gail Eisnitz, Ingrid Newkirk, Susan Roghair, Alex Hershaft, Jim Mason, Richard Schwartz, Rynn Berry, Steve Hindi, Tom Regan, Don Barnes, Ray Greek, and Carol Adams.

For providing me with the tools to become a better, more compassionate person: John Robbins, Jeff Nelson, Harshad Parakh, Eva Jones, Alex Jack, Ruth Heidrich, Pamela Rice, Maynard Clark, Gary Null, Nan Taska, Len Horowitz, Richard Kurtz, and Frances Moore Lappe.

For leading me down the path of activism: Barbara Mullarkey, Betty Martini, Alix Cassaday, Mark Sutton, Pete Hardin, Jeremy Rifkin, Freya and Jay Dinshah, Dave Rietz, Tom Rodgers, Joe Connelly, Jerry Cook, Elliott Katz, and Mike Siegel.

For teaching me about Seventh-day Adventists: David Goswick, who sent to me a copy of *Counsels on Diet and Foods* by Ellen G. White; Tammy and Al Roesch, who, together with their family, shared their home with me for a Sabbath weekend; David Koliadko, M.J. Lewis, and Agatha Thrash, who, with love and passion, continue to instruct me; and Nancy and Jeff Riedesel and Danny Vierra, who continue to promote and spread Ellen G. White's message of health.

For helping with the production of this book: Publisher and friend Rudy Shur of Square One Publishers, who, together with the professional assistance of editors Elaine Kennedy and Marie Caratozzolo, oversaw the production of the book you now hold in your hands.

Finally, for continually nourishing my spirit: Lisa, my loving and supportive wife; Jennifer, Sarah, and Lizzy, my wonderful daughters; and Mom and Dad, my guiding lights.

Preface

*I*n 1994, the U.S. Food and Drug Administration (FDA) approved the use of a genetically engineered growth hormone that is injected into cows for increased milk production. The use of this hormone became an immediate and obvious cause of concern for health advocates. As a scientific researcher and protective parent of three daughters, I began an investigation of genetically modified organisms (GMOs) and their effect on the food industry—primarily on dairy products.

The research of writer Jane Heimlich was inspirational in further arousing my investigative interest. The wife of Dr. Henry Heimlich (originator of the Heimlich Maneuver), Jane is the author of many books on health and nutrition, including the bestseller *What Your Doctor Won't Tell You*. Interestingly, I had met her husband years earlier when he performed life-saving surgery on my father. I was thirteen years old at the time. Thirty-three years later, I was a dinner guest in their home. The simplicity of that evening's meal—freshly baked whole wheat bread, roasted home-grown tomatoes, and a salad served with aged Balsamic vinegar and cold-pressed olive oil made from organic olives—was memorable. It inspired me to forever cross the line from carnivore to vegetarian. A true vegan, I no longer eat animal products. My diet consists entirely of plant foods: fruits, vegetables, nuts, seeds, and grains.

Through my intensive and continued investigation of the

dairy industry and dairy products, I uncovered scientific evidence that shot holes through the National Dairy Board's slogan: "Milk. It does a body good." This belief was, in actuality, one of America's greatest myths. Discovering the little-publicized harmful effects of dairy products on health and wellness prompted me to take action. I wrote two books: *MILK—The Deadly Poison* and *Milk A-Z*. It also propelled me to become a key player in the anti-dairy movement. I have appeared on hundreds of television programs and radio shows, and have been the subject of newspaper and magazine articles, and editorials in dairy industry journals. I've also lectured at countless numbers of colleges and churches, as well as conferences for animal rights groups and industry organizations. I have testified before government agencies, and have been involved with the USDA's Dietary Guidelines Committee.

In April of 2003, I lectured at a Seventh-day Adventist Church (SDA) in Brooklyn, New York. In preparation for the lecture, I read Ellen G. White's *Counsels on Diet and Foods*. I could not put it down. The nutritional advice of the SDA founder paralleled the same principles that I supported. Her nineteenth-century healing words of wisdom sounded like dietary advice offered by great twenty-first century physicians and dietitians. The latter's beliefs are validated by scientific evidence—conclusions demonstrating that nations consuming the greatest amounts of meat and dairy products also have the highest rates of cancer, osteoporosis, heart disease, asthma, and diabetes.

During the early part of my lecture that day, I asked the children, "Who loves ice cream and pizza?" Every hand shot straight up. Having just read White's belief in avoiding the consumption of animal products, I was surprised at this reaction. Although the congregation may have followed a vegetarian diet, it was obvious that they also consumed dairy products. I then asked, "What does the word 'never' mean?" All hands rose again, and I went through the crowd with a microphone, allowing various children to volunteer their answers. One little girl summed up the spirit of "never" by saying, "Never means don't do something, ever." I then read to the congregation the following passage from Ellen G. White's *Counsels on Diet and Foods:*

> "Cheese should *never* be introduced into the stomach;
> it is wholly unfit for food."

When I spoke of Ellen G. White that day, I experienced first-hand the love and adoration felt by the members of the congregation for her, their spiritual leader. As with many important movements, however, certain guidelines had become blurred over time. The flock had drifted somewhat from White's original dietary tenets, which she believed were necessary for promoting good health.

My experience that day inspired me to create this book. In an effort to rediscover Ellen White's pure and simple nutritional philosophy, I have selected 500 quotations from her works that can shed light on her "Garden of Eden" vision. Those following Ellen G. White's teaching will easily digest this new food for thought. Her words will help guide them to attain the promise of better physical and spiritual health.

—Robert Cohen
Editor

Foreword

My experience with Ellen G. White

Ellen G. White was one of the most remarkable women to ever live. Inspired by God, she had a compassion that was never tainted with sentimentalism and insights that were born of the wisdom of ages.

One of the most prolific women writers of all time, Ellen White wrote dozens of books, many pamphlets, and thousands of articles. The sheer variety of topics upon which she wrote—from how to plant a tree to how to build a sterling character to how to administer home remedies to children—outstrips that of any other individual in history. She was a nutritionist with facts as up-to-date as those found in this morning's nutrition journals. Aside from the Bible, her works are the most translated in history.

Throughout history, there have been individuals who have been inspired by God. Ellen White is one of them. In an age of great medical superstition and error, Ellen White included in her writings about medical matters, only that which was factual and accurate, and she acknowledged the source of her wisdom by frequently saying such things as "the Lord showed me," or "I saw it in a vision." In my personal library, there are many books on medical topics. There is not a book that does not contain some difference of opinion from one part of the book to another. One of the remarkable characteristics of Ellen White's writings lies in the consistency and agreement of the material, and we are simply astounded when we come to understand that some of what she wrote was not discovered by medical researchers until the very present decade.

Two great benchmarks are available to the physician upon which to base a judgment—well-done research and divine inspiration. Ellen White was able to sort out from the dark and muddy maze of medical fact and folklore of her age only that which was enduring truth. She was a very capable writer in blending enduring truths with that which was inspired. A student who knows only what White has written and nothing else would be considered highly educated.

My experience with Robert Cohen

I first became acquainted with Robert Cohen a few years ago when he sent me a letter of enquiry concerning his research on artificial milks and their superiority to dairy milk. My own investigation had led me to believe that dairy milk is not only unsafe medically, it is revolting esthetically. With both pen and voice, I have tried to make others aware of the dangers hidden in this innocent looking all-American drink. Robert Cohen is someone with a stronger voice than mine. He is a careful researcher, delightful speaker, and ingenious organizer. The way he has presented the material in this book has further garnered my respect for him as a writer.

What you can expect to get from *God's Nutritionist*

Do not expect to be the same person after reading this book. You will come to know certain practical aspects of the physiology of digestion. You can also expect to be led toward changes in your lifestyle for the betterment of your health. *God's Nutritionist* will enrich your life and ennoble your spirit. After reading it, you will have two new friends: Ellen G. White and Robert Cohen.

—Agatha M. Thrash, MD
Medical Director Emeritus
Uchee Pines Institute

God's Nutritionist

Introduction

I n 1863, Ellen Gould White became one of the spiritual founders and architects of the Seventh-day Adventist (SDA) faith. Believed to be a prophet of God, White was a woman of remarkable spiritual gifts. Today, her followers include some 13 million church members. The essence of Ellen G. White's dietary philosophy on physical and spiritual health is presented in this book in the form of 500 divinely inspired "pearls of wisdom." Each "pearl" was gleaned from letters, speeches, articles, and books that were written by White over her seventy-year career. Eventually, these writings were edited by the trustees of her estate and compiled in the work *Counsels on Diet and Foods*, first published in 1938. Long before America's first fad diet book was written, Ellen G. White recognized the harmful effects of meat and dairy products on the human body, and her beliefs were eventually validated through scientific research. Fascinating excerpts from scientific magazines and peer-reviewed journals, verifying White's inspired beliefs, are presented in this book along with each of her "pearls of wisdom."

Over the years, Ellen G. White has become the most translated author in the history of American literature. During her writing career, she produced 50,000 pages of manuscript, which have been translated into 140 different languages. Many Adventists believe that her writings are just one level below that of the Scriptures.

Born Ellen Harmon on November 26, 1827, she married Preacher James White at seventeen years of age, and gave birth to their first child before her twentieth birthday. At the age of twenty-four, White published her first book in which she disclosed many of her own personal revelations. By age thirty-three, she was mother to four sons. Shortly after the founding of the Seventh-day Adventist Church, she experienced her first vision of the relationship between physical health and spirituality. That vision became one of the cornerstones of the SDA religious credo.

Ellen and James were married for thirty-five years when James died. Ellen continued to write and lecture for an additional thirty-four years until her own death in 1915 at age eighty-seven. Through her passionate mission, some 136,000 Adventists came to believe that she was a messenger of God.

In 1870, White wrote, "Very many animals are sold for the city market known to be diseased by those who have sold them, and those who buy them are not always ignorant of the matter. Especially in larger cities this is practiced to a great extent, and meat eaters know not that they are eating diseased animals." These prophetic words can easily apply to newly emerging diseases that are spread by animals, including Severe Acute Respiratory Syndrome (SARS) and Bovine Spongiform Encephalopathy (BSE), more commonly known as "Mad Cow Disease."

At about the same time that Susan B. Anthony and Elizabeth Cady Stanton were arguing for women's rights, Ellen G. White was advocating for animal rights. When Buffalo Bill was killing thousands of bison to feed railroad workers, Ellen G. White was organizing tens of thousands of people to love animals by not eating them. While General Custer was experiencing his last stand, Ellen G. White was taking a stand for animals that was heard by people throughout the world. To date, her movement has inspired over 13 million followers.

White's dietary advice was combined with her compassion for animals. She wrote, "Animals are often transported long distances and subjected to great suffering in reaching a market.

Taken from the green pastures and traveling for weary miles over the hot, dusty roads, or crowded into filthy cars, feverish and exhausted, often for many hours deprived of food and water, the poor creatures are driven to their death, that human beings may feast on the carcasses." She also wrote, "Some animals that are brought to the slaughter seem to realize by instinct what is to take place, and they become furious, and literally mad. They are killed while in that state, and their flesh is prepared for market. Their meat is poison, and has produced, in those who have eaten it, cramps, convulsions, apoplexy, and sudden death. Yet the cause of all this suffering is not attributed to the meat."

White also warned, "Cheese should never be introduced into the stomach." Through her controversial declaration, "Animals from which milk is obtained are not always healthy. They may be diseased. A cow may be apparently well in the morning, and die before night. Then she was diseased in the morning, and her milk was diseased, but you did not know it," she gained ardent followers. Today's vegans would have applauded statements such as the following one, which was written in 1893: "Especially harmful are the custards and puddings in which milk, eggs, and sugar are the chief ingredients. The use of milk and sugar taken together should be avoided."

White recognized that consumers needed alternatives to the standard American diet. In her millennium address of January 1, 1900, she told thousands of listeners, "The health food business is in need of means and of the active cooperation of our people, that it may accomplish the work it ought to do. Its purpose is to supply the people with food which will take the place of flesh meat, and also milk and butter." Her message to avoid milk included this food for thought, "If for dessert sweet cake is eaten with milk or cream, fermentation will be created in the stomach, and then the weak points of the human organism will tell the story. The brain will be affected by the disturbance in the stomach."

White's inspirations were revealed without the benefit of modern-day scientific peer-reviewed journals, which, by the late

1900s, had cumulatively published thousands of articles supporting the conclusion that adverse effects result from the consumption of milk and dairy products. Scientists living in 1870 did not dream of the existence of bovine growth hormones, nor did they possess the conclusive scientific link between bovine proteins and insulin-dependent diabetes, irritable bowel syndrome, and arthritis. There was little exposure to cancer, heart disease, asthma, and osteoporosis. Their nineteenth-century diets little resembled the foods eaten in our twenty-first century world, in which man has the ability to process foods in factories, add chemicals to emulsify and preserve, and refrigerate those foods to retard spoilage.

White dedicated seventy years of her life to health reform. Her 1883 advice rings true over 100 years later, "Fresh air, exercise, pure water, and clean, sweet premises, are within the reach of all, with but little expense; but drugs are expensive, both in the outlay of means, and the effect produced upon the system."

It is my hope that you, the reader, will use this book as a daily inspiration, or as an uninterrupted reading event that may lead you to a lifestyle change or confirm what you already know: that diet influences every aspect of one's physical, intellectual, and philosophical growth. If Ellen G. White were with us today, her voice, energy, and spirit would still be leading us on a way of life that is in tune with nature—in tune with God. Born long before her time, she was truly an amazing woman whose message is as relevant now as it was then. Here then are 500 pearls of wisdom from Ellen G. White to guide and inspire us all.

"God said, 'Behold, I have given you every seed bearing plant on the face of the earth, and every tree that has seed bearing fruit. It shall be to you for food.'"

Genesis 1:29

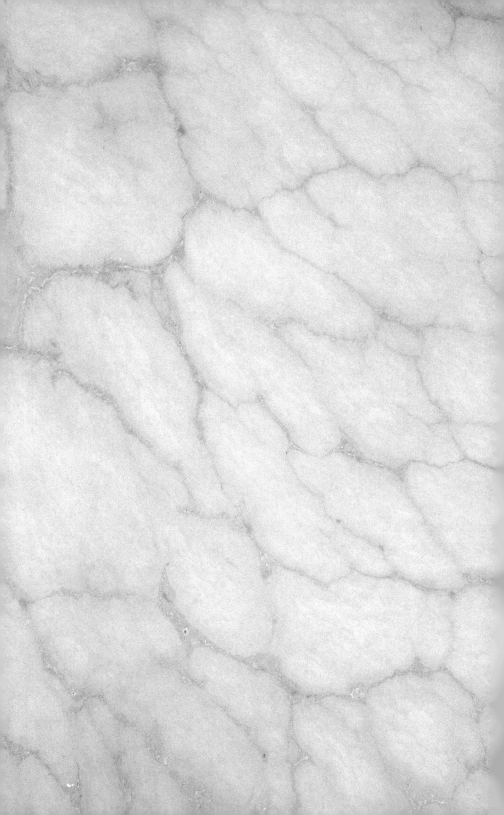

1

I am so thankful to God that when Adam lost his Eden home, the Lord did not cut off the supply of fruit. *(1857 Letter)*

2

*I*n order to know what are the best foods, we must study God's original plan for man's diet. He who created man and who understands his needs appointed Adam his food. "Behold," He said, "I have given you every herb yielding seed,. . . . and every tree, in which is the fruit of a tree yielding seed; to you it shall be for food." Upon leaving Eden to gain his livelihood by tilling the earth under the curse of sin, man received permission to eat also "the herb of the field." *(Ministry of Healing, 1905)*

3

*G*rains, fruits, nuts, and vegetables constitute the diet chosen for us by our Creator. These foods prepared in as simple and natural a manner as possible, are the most healthful and nourishing. They impart a strength, a power of endurance, and a vigor of intellect, that are not afforded by a more complex and stimulating diet. *(Ministry of Healing, 1905)*

4

*M*eat is not essential for health or strength, else the Lord made a mistake when He provided food for Adam and Eve before their fall. All the elements of nutrition are contained in the fruits, vegetables, and grains. *(Review and Herald, May 8, 1883)*

5

God has, with a lavish hand, provided us with rich and varied bounties for our sustenance and enjoyment.
(Testimonies for the Church, Volume 4, 1876)

6

Those who eat flesh are but eating grains and vegetables at second hand; for the animal receives from these things the nutrition that produces growth. The life that was in the grains and vegetables passes into the eater. We receive it by eating the flesh of the animal. How much better to get it direct, by eating the food that God provided for our use! *(Ministry of Healing, 1905)*

7

Overeating has a worse effect upon the system than overworking; the energies of the soul are more effectually prostrated by intemperate eating than by intemperate working.
(Testimonies, Volume 2, 1870)

8

God gave our first parents the food He designed that the race should eat. It was contrary to His plan to have the life of any creature taken. There was to be no death in Eden. The fruit of the trees in the garden, was the food man's wants required.
(Spiritual Gifts, Volume 4, 1856)

"Incidence of lung and colorectal cancer is lower in vegetarians than in non-vegetarians."

Cancer incidence among California Seventh-day Adventists, 1976–1982. *American Journal of Clinical Nutrition*, 1994; 59 (supplement):1136S–1142S.

9

God provided fruit in its natural state for our first parents. God is working in behalf of His people. He does not desire them to be without resources. He is bringing them back to the diet originally given to man. Their diet is to consist of the foods made from the materials He has provided. The materials principally used in these foods will be fruits and grains and nuts, but various roots will also be used. *(Testimonies, Volume 4, 1890)*

"Western vegetarians have significantly lower average serum total cholesterol concentrations, body mass index, and blood pressure, all well-established diet-related risk factors for coronary heart disease. Of particular interest is that the lower average serum total cholesterol concentration would be expected to result in an approximately 25% reduction in mortality from coronary heart disease among vegetarians compared with non-vegetarians."

Nutrition, May, 2003, Volume 19, Issue 3, 285–289

10

Again and again I have been shown that God is bringing His people back to His original design, that is, not to subsist upon the flesh of dead animals. He would have us teach people a better way . . . If meat is discarded, if the taste is not educated in that direction, if a liking for fruits and grains is encouraged, it will soon be as God in the beginning designed it should be. No meat will be used by His people. *(1884 Letter)*

11

A failure to care for the living machinery is an insult to the Creator. There are divinely appointed rules which if observed will keep human beings from disease and premature death. *(1901 Letter)*

12

*I*t is a mistake to suppose that muscular strength depends on the use of animal food. The needs of the system can be better supplied, and more vigorous health can be enjoyed, without its use. *(Ministry of Healing, 1905)*

13

*I*f ever there was a time when the diet should be of the most simple kind, it is now. *(Testimonies, Volume 2, 1869)*

14

*M*any articles of food which a few years ago were regarded as expensive luxuries, are now within the reach of all as foods for everyday use. This is especially the case with dried and canned fruits. *(Ministry of Healing, 1905)*

15

*T*o keep the body in a healthy condition, in order that all parts of the living machinery may act harmoniously, should be a study of our life. The children of God cannot glorify Him with sickly bodies or dwarfed minds. Those who indulge in any species of intemperance, either in eating or drinking, waste their physical energies and weaken moral power. *(Christian Temperance and Bible Hygiene, 1890)*

16

*K*nowledge must be gained in regard to how to eat, and drink, and dress so as to preserve health. Sickness is caused by violating the laws of health; it is the result of violating nature's law. *(Testimonies, Volume 3, 1872)*

"Total serum cholesterol and low-density lipoprotein cholesterol levels are usually lower in vegetarians, but high-density lipoprotein cholesterol and triglyceride levels vary depending on the type of vegetarian diet followed."

Journal of the American Dietetic Association, November 1997, 97(1) citing the *American Journal of Clinical Nutrition,* 1994; 59:103–109

17

*E*very man has the opportunity, to a great extent, of making himself whatever he chooses to be. The blessings of this life, and also of the immortal state, are within his reach. He may build up a character of solid worth, gaining new strength at every step. He may advance daily in knowledge and wisdom, conscious of new delights as he progresses, adding virtue to virtue, grace to grace. His faculties will improve by use; the more wisdom he gains, the greater will be his capacity for acquiring. His intelligence, knowledge, and virtue will thus develop into greater strength and more perfect symmetry. *(Christian Temperance and Bible Hygiene, 1890)*

18

*H*ealth is a treasure. Of all temporal possessions it is the most precious. Wealth, learning, and honor are dearly purchased at the loss of the vigor of health. None of these can secure happiness, if health is lacking. *(Christian Temperance and Bible Hygiene, 1890)*

19

*I*n order to preserve health, temperance in all things is necessary,—temperance in labor, temperance in eating and drinking. *(Counsels on Health, 1890)*

20

Only when we are intelligent in regard to the principles of healthful living, can we be fully aroused to see the evils resulting from improper diet. *(Testimonies, Volume 9, 1909)*

"Vegetarian diets offer disease protection benefits because of their lower saturated fat, cholesterol, and animal protein content and often higher concentration of folate (which reduces serum homocysteine levels), antioxidants such as vitamins C and E, carotenoids, and phytochemicals."

Journal of the American Dietetic Association, 1995; 95:180–189

21

Luxurious food and wine were prohibited, in order to promote physical vigor, fortitude, and firmness. *(Christian Temperance and Bible Hygiene, 1890)*

22

Our danger is not from scarcity, but from abundance. We are constantly tempted to excess. *(Christian Temperance and Bible Hygiene, 1890)*

23

Those who have received instruction regarding the evils of the use of flesh foods, tea and coffee, and rich and unhealthful food preparations, and who are determined to make a covenant with God by sacrifice, will not continue to indulge their appetite for food that they know to be unhealthful. *(Testimonies, Volume 9, 1909)*

24

We have been given the work of advancing health reform.
(1902 Letter)

25

God will cooperate with His children in preserving their
health, if they eat with care, refusing to put unnecessary burdens
on the stomach. He has graciously made the path of nature sure
and safe, wide enough for all who walk in it. He has given for
our sustenance the wholesome and health-giving productions of
the earth. *(1902 Letter)*

26

Excessive indulgence in eating, drinking, sleeping, or seeing,
is sin. The harmonious healthy action of all the powers of body
and mind results in happiness; and the more elevated and refined
the powers, the more pure and unalloyed the happiness.
(Testimonies, Volume 4, 1880)

"Eating a diet rich in plant foods, in the form of fruits, vegetables, and
whole-grain cereals, probably remains the best option for reducing the
risk of colon cancer, and for more general health protection."

The Lancet, May 3, 2003, Volume 361, p 1448

27

A large proportion of all the infirmities that afflict the
human family, are the results of their own wrong habits. *(Health
Reformer, March, 1878)*

28

*I*t is a duty to know how to preserve the body in the very best condition of health, and it is a sacred duty to live up to the light which God has graciously given. *(Testimonies, Volume 2, 1868)*

29

*C*hange your course of living, your eating, your drinking, and your working. While you pursue the course you have been following for years, you cannot clearly discern sacred and eternal things. Your sensibilities are blunted, and your intellect beclouded. You have not been growing in grace and in the knowledge of the truth as was your privilege. You have not been increasing in spirituality, but growing more and more darkened. *(Testimonies, Volume 2, 1868)*

30

*G*od requires of His people continual advancement. We need to learn that indulged appetite is the greatest hindrance to mental improvement and soul sanctification. With all our profession of health reform, many of us eat improperly. *(Testimonies, Volume 9, 1909)*

31

*O*ften the stomach is overburdened with food which is seldom as plain and simple as that eaten at home, where the amount of exercise taken is double or treble. This causes the mind to be in such a lethargy that it is difficult to appreciate eternal things. *(Testimonies, Volume 5, 1882)*

"Using a macrobiotic diet emphasizing whole grains, vegetables, and legumes while avoiding dairy products and most meats, nine men with prostate cancer had an average survival of 228 months, compared to 72 months for a matched group of men using no special diet."

Journal of the American College of Nutrition, 1993; 12:209–26

32

The most precious words may be heard and not appreciated, because the mind is confused by an improper diet. *(Ministry of Healing, 1905)*

33

You need clear, energetic minds, in order to appreciate the exalted character of the truth, to value the atonement, and to place the right estimate upon eternal things. *(Testimonies, Volume 2, 1868)*

34

Some are indulging lustful appetite, which wars against the soul, and is a constant hindrance to their spiritual advancement. They constantly bear an accusing conscience, and if straight truths are talked, they are prepared to be offended. They are self-condemned, and feel that subjects have been purposely selected to touch their case. They feel grieved and injured, and withdraw themselves from the assemblies of the saints. They forsake the assembling of themselves together, for then their consciences are not so disturbed. *(Testimonies, Volume 1, 1867)*

35

*B*utter and meat stimulate. These have injured the stomach and perverted the taste. The sensitive nerves of the brain have been benumbed, and the animal appetite strengthened at the expense of the moral and intellectual faculties. *(Testimonies, Volume 2, 1870)*

36

*A*nything that lessens physical strength enfeebles the mind, and makes it less capable of discriminating between right and wrong. We become less capable of choosing the good, and have less strength of will to do that which we know to be right. *(Christ's Object Lessons, 1900)*

"Well-planned vegan diets are appropriate for all stages of the life cycle, including during pregnancy and lactation. Appropriately planned vegan and lacto-ovo-vegetarian diets satisfy nutrient needs of infants, children, and adolescents and promote normal growth."
Journal of the American Dietetic Association, November 1997, 97(1) citing the *American Journal of Clinical Nutrition, 1994; 59 (suppl):1176S–1181S.*

37

*T*hose who eat and work intemperately and irrationally, talk and act irrationally. An intemperate man cannot be a patient man. It is not necessary to drink alcoholic liquors in order to be intemperate. The sin of intemperate eating, eating too frequently, too much, and of rich, unwholesome food, destroys the healthy action of the digestive organs, affects the brain, and perverts the judgment, preventing rational, calm, healthy thinking and acting. *(Testimonies, Volume 1, 1867)*

38

*P*hysical habits have a great deal to do with the success of every individual. The more careful you are in your diet, the more simple and un-stimulating the food that sustains the body in its harmonious action, the more clear will be your conception of duty. There needs to be a careful review of every habit, every practice, lest a morbid condition of the body shall cast a cloud upon everything. *(1898 Letter)*

39

*T*he use of unnatural stimulants is destructive to health and has a benumbing influence upon the brain, making it impossible to appreciate eternal things. *(Testimonies, Volume 1, 1867)*

40

*T*here are but few as yet who are aroused sufficiently to understand how much their habits of diet have to do with their health, their characters, their usefulness in this world, and their eternal destiny. *(Testimonies, Volume 1, 1867)*

41

*O*ur race is in a deplorable condition, suffering from disease of every description. Many have inherited disease, and are great sufferers because of the wrong habits of their parents; and yet they pursue the same wrong course in regard to themselves and their children which was pursued toward them. They are ignorant in regard to themselves. They are sick and do not know that their own wrong habits are causing them immense suffering. *(Testimonies, Volume 1, 1867)*

"Vegan diets can meet the nutrient and energy needs of pregnant women. Birth weights of infants born to well nourished vegetarian women have been shown to be similar to birth-weight norms and to birth weights of infants of non vegetarians."

Pediatrics, 1989; 84

42

*f*ny unhealthful habit will produce an unhealthful condition in the system, and the delicate, living machinery of the stomach will be injured, and will not be able to do its work properly. The diet has much to do with the disposition to enter into temptation and commit sin. *(Manuscript Files, 1901)*

43

The indulgence of appetite affects them in all the relations of life. It is seen in their family, in their church, in the prayer meeting, and in the conduct of their children. It has been the curse of their lives. You cannot make them understand the truths for these last days. *(Testimonies, Volume 2, 1870)*

44

Those who permit themselves to become slaves to a gluttonous appetite, often go still farther, and debase themselves by indulging their corrupt passions, which have become excited by intemperance in eating and in drinking. They give loose rein to their debasing passions, until health and intellect greatly suffer. The reasoning faculties are, in a great measure, destroyed by evil habits. *(Spiritual Gifts, Book 4, 1867)*

45

*A*nd if the food is not the most healthful, the effects will be still more injurious. Any habit which does not promote healthful action in the human system, degrades the higher and nobler faculties. Wrong habits of eating and drinking lead to errors in thought and action. Indulgence of appetite strengthens the animal propensities, giving them the ascendancy over the mental and spiritual powers. *(Review and Herald, January 25, 1881)*

46

*T*he gospel of health has able advocates, but their work has been made very hard because so many ministers, presidents of conferences, and others in positions of influence, have failed to give the question of health reform its proper attention. They have not recognized it in its relation to the work of the message as the right arm of the body. *(Testimonies, Volume 6, 1900)*

"Certified death rates from coronary heart disease (CHD) are positively correlated country-by-country with milk consumption, particularly with that of the non-fat portion of milk."

International Journal of Cardiology, February 2003, Vol 87, Issue 2/3

47

*L*et those who advocate health reform strive earnestly to make it all that they claim it is. Let them discard everything detrimental to health. Use simple, wholesome food. Fruit is excellent, and saves much cooking. Discard rich pastries, cakes, desserts, and the other dishes prepared to tempt the appetite. Eat fewer kinds of food at one meal, and eat with thanksgiving. *(1902 Letter)*

48

They should be temperate in eating; rich and luxurious food should find no place upon their tables; and when the brain is constantly taxed, and there is a lack of physical exercise, they should eat sparingly, even of plain food. *(Testimonies, Volume 4, 1880)*

49

What a pity it is that often, when the greatest self-denial should be exercised, the stomach is crowded with a mass of unhealthful food, which lies there to decompose. The affliction of the stomach affects the brain. *(Manuscript Files, 1901)*

50

Many marvel that the human race have so degenerated, physically, mentally, and morally. They do not understand that it is the violation of God's constitution and laws, and the violation of the laws of health, that has produced this sad degeneracy. *(Spiritual Gifts, 1864)*

51

No man can become a successful workman in spiritual things until he observes strict temperance in his dietetic habits. *(Spiritual Gifts, Undated)*

52

Meat should not be placed before our children. Its influence is to excite and strengthen the lower passions, and has a tendency to deaden the moral powers. *(Testimonies, Volume 2, 1869)*

53

Grains and fruits prepared free from grease, and in as natural a condition as possible, should be the food for the tables of all who claim to be preparing for translation to heaven. *(Testimonies, Volume 2, 1869)*

54

You place upon your table food which taxes the digestive organs, excites the animal passions, and weakens the moral and intellectual faculties. Rich food and flesh meats are no benefit to you. *(Testimonies, Volume 2, 1869)*

"Vegetarians tend to have a lower incidence of hypertension than non-vegetarians."

Journal of the American Dietetic Association, November 1997, 97(1) citing the *American Journal of Clinical Nutrition,* 1994; 59 (suppl):1130–1135

55

Abstain from fleshly lusts which war against the soul. You need to practice temperance in all things. Here is a cross which you have shunned. To confine yourself to a simple diet, which will preserve you in the best of condition of health, is a task to you. *(Testimonies, Volume 2, 1868)*

56

My dear friends, instead of taking a course to baffle disease, you are petting it and yielding to its power. You should avoid the use of drugs, and carefully observe the laws of health. *(Testimonies, Volume 5, 1885)*

"At least 50% of all children in the United States are allergic to milk, many undiagnosed. Dairy products are the leading cause of food allergy, often revealed by constipation, diarrhea, and fatigue. Many cases of asthma and sinus infections are reported to be relieved and even eliminated by cutting out dairy."

Frank Oski, M.D., Chief of Pediatrics at Johns Hopkins Medical School
Natural Health, July, 1994

57

Persons who have accustomed themselves to a rich, highly stimulating diet, have an unnatural taste, and they cannot at once relish food that is plain and simple. It will take time for the taste to become natural, and for the stomach to recover from the abuse it has suffered. But those who persevere in the use of wholesome food will, after a time, find it palatable. Its delicate and delicious flavors will be appreciated, and it will be eaten with greater enjoyment than can be derived from unwholesome dainties. And the stomach, in a healthy condition, neither fevered nor overtaxed, can readily perform its task. *(Ministry of Healing, 1905)*

58

Eating, drinking, and dressing all have a direct bearing upon our spiritual advancement. *(Youth Instructor, May 31, 1894)*

59

A reform in eating would be a saving of expense and labor. The wants of a family can be easily supplied that is satisfied with plain, wholesome diet. Rich food breaks down the healthy organs of body and mind. *(Spiritual Gifts, Volume 4, 1864)*

60

$\mathcal{W}$e are all to consider that there is to be no extravagance in any line. We must be satisfied with pure, simple food, prepared in a simple manner. This should be the diet of high and low. Adulterated substances are to be avoided. *(1905 Letter)*

61

$\mathcal{H}$urtful food and drinks are partaken of in such a measure as to greatly tax the organs of digestion. The vital forces are called into unnecessary action in the disposal of it, which produces exhaustion, and greatly disturbs the circulation of the blood, and, as a result, want of vital energy is felt throughout the system. *(How to Live, Book 1, 1865)*

62

$\mathcal{I}$n order to have good health, we must have good blood; for the blood is the current of life. It repairs waste, and nourishes the body. When supplied with the proper food elements and when cleansed and vitalized by contact with pure air, it carries life and vigor to every part of the system. The more perfect the circulation, the better will this work be accomplished. *(Ministry of Healing, 1905)*

"Dietary fat during childhood may be more life-threatening than was originally suspected . . . Overweight children are usually the victims of the dietary habits of the adult members of the family . . . Reducing dietary fat to levels necessary to the control of cholesterol cannot be achieved if a child drinks whole milk or eats cheese."

Charles Attwood, M.D., *Dr. Attwood's Low-Fat Prescription for Kids*

63

*M*any have inquired of me, What course shall I take best to preserve my health? My answer is, Cease to transgress the laws of your being; cease to gratify a depraved appetite, eat simple food, dress healthfully, which will require modest simplicity, work healthfully, and you will not be sick. *(Health Reformer, August, 1865)*

64

*I*f men were today simple in their habits, living in harmony with nature's laws, there would be an abundant supply for all the needs of the human family. There would be fewer imaginary wants, and more opportunity to work in God's ways. *(Testimonies, Volume 6, 1900)*

65

*T*hose who entertain visitors, should have wholesome, nutritious food, from fruits, grains, and vegetables, prepared in a simple, tasteful manner. Such cooking will require but little extra labor or expense, and, partaken of in moderate quantities, will not injure any one. *(How to Live, Book 1, 1865)*

66

*I*n the use of foods, we should exercise good, sound common sense. When we find that a certain food does not agree with us, we need not write letters of inquiry to learn the cause of the disturbance. Change the diet; use less of some foods; try other preparations. Soon we shall know the effect that certain combinations have on us. *(Testimonies, Volume 7, 1902)*

67

The true fasting which should be recommended to all, is abstinence from every stimulating kind of food, and the proper use of wholesome, simple food, which God has provided in abundance. *(1896 Letter)*

"The beef industry has contributed to more American deaths than all the wars of this century, all natural disasters, and all automobile accidents combined. If beef is your idea of real food for real people, you'd better live real close to a real good hospital."

Neal Barnard, M.D., Physicians Committee for Responsible Medicine

68

Because it is wrong to eat merely to gratify perverted taste, it does not follow that we should be indifferent in regard to our food. It is a matter of the highest importance. No one should adopt an impoverished diet. *(Manuscript Files, 1901)*

69

Not all foods wholesome in themselves are equally suited to our needs under all circumstances. Care should be taken in the selection of food. *(Ministry of Healing, 1905)*

70

Some of our people conscientiously abstain from eating improper food, and at the same time neglect to eat the food that would supply the elements necessary for the proper sustenance of the body. *(1902 Letter)*

71

Some householders stint the family table in order to provide expensive entertainment for visitors. This is unwise. In the entertainment of guests there should be greater simplicity. Let the needs of the family have first attention. *(Ministry of Healing, 1905)*

72

In grains, fruits, vegetables, and nuts are to be found all the food elements that we need. If we will come to the Lord in simplicity of mind, He will teach us how to prepare wholesome food free from the taint of flesh meat. *(Manuscript Files, 1906)*

73

Let us make intelligent advancement in simplifying our diet. In the providence of God, every country produces articles of food containing the nourishment necessary for the up-building of the system. These may be made into healthful, appetizing dishes. *(1902 Letter)*

"With the exception of tobacco consumption, diet is probably the most important factor in the etiology of human cancer."

Toxicology, December, 2002, Volume 181–182

74

The foods used should correspond to the climate. Some foods suitable for one country would not do at all in another place. *(1901 Letter)*

75

We do not mark out any precise line to be followed in diet; but we do say that in countries where there are fruits, grain, and nuts in abundance, flesh food is not the right food for God's people. *(Testimonies, Volume 9, 1909)*

76

God has given us an ample variety of healthful foods, and each person should choose from it the things that experience and sound judgment prove to be best suited to his own necessities. *(Ministry of Healing, 1905)*

77

Wherever dried fruits, such as raisins, prunes, apples, pears, peaches, and apricots, are obtainable at moderate prices, it will be found that they can be used as staple articles of diet much more freely than is customary, with the best results to the health and vigor of all classes of workers. *(Ministry of Healing, 1905)*

78

It is the Lord's design that in every place men and women shall be encouraged to develop their talents by preparing healthful foods from the natural products of their own section of the country. If they look to God, exercising their skill and ingenuity under the guidance of His Spirit, they will learn how to prepare natural products into healthful foods. Thus they will be able to teach the poor how to provide themselves with foods that will take the place of flesh meats. Those thus helped can in turn instruct others. *(Testimonies, Volume 7, 1902)*

"In a controlled trial, 21 strict vegetarians were studied prospectively for eight weeks: a two-week control period of the usual vegetarian diet was followed by four weeks, during which 250 g of beef was added isocalorically to the daily vegetarian diet and then by two weeks of the control diet. Plasma total cholesterol rose significantly by 19% at the end of the meat eating period."

Journal of the American Medical Association, 1981 Aug 7; 246(6):640

79

Respect paid to the proper treatment of the stomach will be rewarded in clearness of thought and strength of mind. Your digestive organs will not be prematurely worn out to testify against you. *(1908 Letter)*

80

The Lord will teach many in all parts of the world to combine fruits, grains, and vegetables into foods that will sustain life and will not bring disease. Those who have never seen the recipes for making the health foods now on the market, will work intelligently, experimenting with the food productions of the earth, and will be given light regarding the use of these productions. The Lord will show them what to do. He who gives skill and understanding to His people in one part of the world will give skill and understanding to His people in other parts of the world. It is His design that the food treasures of each country shall be so prepared that they can be used in the countries for which they are suited. As God gave manna from heaven to sustain the children of Israel, so He will now give His people in different places skill and wisdom to use the productions of these countries in preparing foods to take the place of meat. *(Testimonies, Volume 7, 1902)*

81

*I*n warm, heating climates, there should be given to the worker, in whatever line of work he is to do, less work than in a more bracing climate. The less sugar introduced into the food in its preparation, the less difficulty will be experienced because of the heat of the climate. *(1898 Letter)*

82

*E*xercise aids the dyspeptic by giving the digestive organs a healthy tone. To engage in deep study or violent exercise immediately after eating, hinders the digestive process; for the vitality of the system, which is needed to carry on the work of digestion, is called away to other parts. But a short walk after a meal, with the head erect and the shoulders back, exercising moderately, is a great benefit. The mind is diverted from self to the beauties of nature. The less the attention is called to the stomach, the better. If you are in constant fear that your food will hurt you, it most assuredly will. Forget your troubles; think of something cheerful. *(Christian Temperance and Bible Hygiene, 1890)*

83

*O*ften this intemperance is felt at once in the form of headache, indigestion, and colic. A load has been placed upon the stomach that it cannot care for, and a feeling of oppression comes. The head is confused, the stomach is in rebellion. But these results do not always follow overeating. In some cases the stomach is paralyzed. No sensation of pain is felt, but the digestive organs lose their vital force. The foundation of the human machinery is gradually undermined, and life is rendered very unpleasant. *(1896 Letter)*

> "Milk and milk products gave the highest correlation coefficient to heart disease, while sugar, animal proteins and animal fats came in second, third, and fourth, respectively."
>
> *Medical Hypothesis*, 7:907–918, 1981

84

There are large blood vessels in the limbs for the purpose of distributing the life-giving current to all parts of the body. The fire you kindle in your stomach is making your brain like a heated furnace. Eat much more sparingly, and eat simple food, which does not require heavy seasoning. *(1908 Letter)*

85

What influence does overeating have upon the stomach? It becomes debilitated, the digestive organs are weakened, and disease, with all its train of evils, is brought on as the result. If persons were diseased before, they thus increase the difficulties upon them, and lessen their vitality every day they live. They call their vital powers into unnecessary action to take care of the food that they place in their stomachs. *(Testimonies, Volume 2, 1870)*

86

My brother, you have much to learn. You indulge your appetite by eating more food than your system can convert into good blood. It is sin to be intemperate in the quantity of food eaten, even if the quality is unobjectionable. Many feel that if they do not eat meat and the grosser articles of food, they may eat of simple food until they cannot well eat more. This is a mistake. *(Testimonies, Volume 2, 1870)*

87

*M*asticate slowly, and allow the saliva to mingle with the food. The more liquid there is taken into the stomach with the meals, the more difficult it is for the food to digest; for the liquid must first be absorbed. *(Counsels on Health, 1890)*

"Mortality from coronary artery disease is lower in vegetarians than in non vegetarians."

British Medical Journal, 1994; 308

88

*M*any professed health reformers are nothing less than gluttons. They lay upon the digestive organs so great a burden that the vitality of the system is exhausted in the effort to dispose of it. It also has a depressing influence upon the intellect; for the brain nerve power is called upon to assist the stomach in its work. *(Testimonies, Volume 2, 1870)*

89

I told them that the preparation of their food was wrong, and that living principally on soups and coffee and bread was not health reform; that so much liquid taken into the stomach was not healthful, and that all who subsisted on such a diet placed a great tax upon the kidneys, and so much watery substance debilitated the stomach. I was thoroughly convinced that many in the establishment were suffering with indigestion because of eating this kind of food. The digestive organs were enfeebled and the blood impoverished. Their breakfast consisted of coffee and bread with the addition of prune sauce. This was not healthful. *(1887 Letter)*

90

The influence of pure, fresh air is to cause the blood to circulate healthfully through the system. It refreshes the body, and tends to render it strong and healthy, while at the same time its influence is decidedly felt upon the mind, imparting a degree of composure and serenity. It excites the appetite, and renders the digestion of food more perfect, and induces sound and sweet sleep. *(Testimonies, Volume 1, 1868)*

91

The lungs should be allowed the greatest freedom possible. Their capacity is developed by free action; it diminishes if they are cramped and compressed. Hence the ill effects of the practice so common, especially in sedentary pursuits, of stooping at one's work. In this position it is impossible to breathe deeply. Superficial breathing soon becomes a habit, and the lungs lose their power to expand A similar effect is produced by tight lacing. Thus an insufficient supply of oxygen is received. The blood moves sluggishly. The waste, poisonous matter, which should be thrown off in the exhalations from the lungs, is retained, and the blood becomes impure. Not only the lungs, but the stomach, liver, and brain are affected. The skin becomes sallow, digestion is retarded; the heart is depressed; the brain is clouded; the thoughts are confused; gloom settles upon the spirits; the whole system becomes depressed and inactive, and peculiarly susceptible to disease. *(Ministry of Healing, 1905)*

"Type 2 diabetes mellitus is less likely to be a cause of death in vegetarians than non vegetarians."

American Journal of Clinical Nutrition, 1988; 48 (suppl)

92

*M*y brother, your brain is benumbed. A man who disposes of the quantity of food that you do, should be a laboring man. Exercise is important to digestion, and to a healthy condition of body and mind. You need physical exercise. You move and act as if you were wooden, as though you had no elasticity. Healthy, active exercise is what you need. This will invigorate the mind. *(1901 Letter)*

93

*H*ot drinks are not required, except as a medicine. The stomach is greatly injured by a large quantity of hot food and hot drink. Thus the throat and digestive organs, and through them the other organs of the body, are enfeebled. *(1901 Letter)*

94

*I*n order to secure healthy digestion, food should be eaten slowly. Those who wish to avoid dyspepsia, and those who realize their obligation to keep all their powers in a condition which will enable them to render the best service to God, will do well to remember this. If your time to eat is limited, do not bolt your food, but eat less, and masticate slowly. The benefit derived from food does not depend so much on the quantity eaten as on its thorough digestion; nor the gratification of taste so much on the amount of food swallowed as on the length of time it remains in the mouth. Those who are excited, anxious, or in a hurry, would do well not to eat until they have found rest or relief; for the vital powers, already severely taxed, cannot supply the necessary digestive fluids. *(Counsels on Health, 1890)*

> "How good it is to be well-fed, healthy, and kind all at the same time."
>
> Henry J. Heimlich, M.D.

95

*M*any do not see the importance of having land to cultivate, and of raising fruit and vegetables, that their tables may be supplied with these things. *(1904 Letter)*

96

*F*ood should not be eaten very hot or very cold. If food is cold, the vital force of the stomach is drawn upon in order to warm it before digestion can take place. Cold drinks are injurious for the same reason; while the free use of hot drinks is debilitating. *(Ministry of Healing, 1890)*

97

*I*f we would work for the restoration of health, it is necessary to restrain the appetite, to eat slowly, and only a limited variety at one meal. This instruction needs to be repeated frequently. It is not in harmony with the principles of health reform to have so many different dishes at one meal. *(1908 Letter)*

98

*F*ood should be eaten slowly, and should be thoroughly masticated. This is necessary, in order that the saliva may be properly mixed with the food, and the digestive fluids be called into action. *(Ministry of Healing, 1890)*

99

I am instructed to say to the workers in our sanitariums and to the teachers and students in our schools that there is need of guarding ourselves upon the point of appetite. There is danger of becoming lax in this respect, and of letting our individual cares and responsibilities so absorb our time that we shall not take time to eat as we should. My message to you is, Take time to eat, and do not crowd into the stomach a great variety of foods at one meal. To eat hurriedly of several kinds of food at a meal is a serious mistake. *(1898 Letter)*

100

*I*t is impossible to prescribe by weight the quantity of food which should be eaten. It is not advisable to follow this process, for by so doing the mind becomes self-centered. Eating and drinking become altogether too much a matter of thought. There are many who have carried a heavy weight of responsibility as to the quantity and quality of food best adapted to nourish the system. Some, especially dyspeptics, have worried so much in regard to their bill of fare that they have not taken sufficient food to nourish the system. They have done great injury to the house they live in, and we fear have spoiled themselves for this life. *(1900 Letter)*

101

*D*o not have too great a variety at a meal; three or four dishes are a plenty. At the next meal you can have a change. The cook should tax her inventive powers to vary the dishes she prepares for the table, and the stomach should not be compelled to take the same kinds of food meal after meal. *(Review and Herald, July 29, 1884)*

102

*A*nother serious evil is eating at improper times, as after violent or excessive exercise, when one is much exhausted or heated. Immediately after eating there is a strong draft upon the nervous energies; and when mind or body is heavily taxed just before or just after eating, digestion is hindered. When one is excited, anxious, or hurried, it is better not to eat until rest or relief is found. *(1898 Letter)*

103

*T*here should not be many kinds at any one meal, but all meals should not be composed of the same kinds of food without variation. Food should be prepared with simplicity, yet with a nicety which will invite the appetite. *(Testimonies, Volume 2, 1868)*

"Vegetarians often have lower mortality rates from several chronic degenerative diseases than do non vegetarians."

British Medical Journal, 1996; 313

104

*G*reat care should be taken when the change is made from a flesh meat to a vegetarian diet to supply the table with wisely prepared, well-cooked articles of food. *(Manuscript Files, 1897)*

105

*I*t would be much better to eat only two or three different kinds of food at a meal than to load the stomach with many varieties. *(1896 Letter)*

106

The stomach is closely related to the brain; and when the stomach is diseased, the nerve power is called from the brain to the aid of the weakened digestive organs. When these demands are too frequent, the brain becomes congested. When the brain is constantly taxed, and there is lack of physical exercise, even plain food should be eaten sparingly. *(Ministry of Healing, 1905)*

"A vegetarian diet can prevent 97% of coronary occlusions."

Journal of the American Medical Association, 179:134–135, 1961

107

Many are made sick by the indulgence of their appetite. So many varieties are introduced into the stomach that fermentation is the result. This condition brings on acute disease, and death frequently follows. *(Manuscript Files, 1897)*

108

The variety of food at one meal causes unpleasantness, and destroys the good which each article, if taken alone, would do the system. This practice causes constant suffering, and often death. *(1896 Letter)*

109

Another cause, both of ill health and of inefficiency in labor, is indigestion. It is impossible for the brain to do its best work when the digestive powers are abused. Many eat hurriedly of various kinds of food, which set up a war in the stomach, and thus confuse the brain. *(Gospel Workers, 1892)*

110

*I*f your work is sedentary, take exercise every day, and at each meal eat only two or three kinds of simple food, taking no more of these than will satisfy the demands of hunger. *(1896 Letter)*

111

*T*here should not be a great variety at any one meal, for this encourages overeating, and causes indigestion. If the digestion is feeble, the use of both will often cause distress, and inability to put forth mental effort. It is better to have the fruit at one meal, and the vegetables at another. The meals should be varied. The same dishes, prepared in the same way, should not appear on the table meal after meal and day after day. The meals are eaten with greater relish, and the system is better nourished, when the food is varied. *(Ministry of Healing, 1905)*

"In Michigan and several other areas, Diphyllobothrium latum, the fish tapeworm, has been identified in man. Opportunity for infection occurs when undercooked fish is eaten. A 51year-old man passed a long, whitish string which he took to his physician. He had had no bowel complaints, but reported a fishing trip to the Northwest area eleven months before. The fish tapeworm normally lives in the small intestine of fish in subarctic and temperate regions. It is the largest tapeworm found in man. It competes with the host for nutrients, which is the major cause for disability produced in man. Especially notable is megaloblastic anemia due to vitamin B-12 deficiency since the tapeworm inhabits the parts of the small bowel where B-12 is absorbed. Numbness of the extremities is the most common complaint, along with fatigue, weakness, and dizziness. All of these are vague and non-specific complaints and can go on for years before the appropriate diagnosis is suspected."

The Animal Connection, Agatha Thrash, M.D. and Calvin Thrash, M.D., p. 8

112

*I*t is not well to take a great variety of foods at one meal. When fruit and bread, together with a variety of other foods that do not agree, are crowded into the stomach at one meal, what can we expect but that a disturbance will be created? *(Manuscript Files, 1897)*

113

*D*isturbance is created by improper combinations of food; fermentation sets in; the blood is contaminated and the brain confused. The habit of overeating, or of eating too many kinds of food at one meal, frequently causes dyspepsia. Serious injury is thus done to the delicate digestive organs. In vain the stomach protests, and appeals to the brain to reason from cause to effect. The excessive amount of food eaten, or the improper combination, does its injurious work. In vain do disagreeable premonitions give warning. Suffering is the consequence. Disease takes the place of health. *(Testimonies, Volume 7, 1902)*

114

*W*e must care for the digestive organs, and not force upon them a great variety of food. He who gorges himself with many kinds of food at a meal is doing himself injury. It is more important that we eat that which will agree with us than that we taste of every dish that may be placed before us. There is no door in our stomach by which we can look in and see what is going on; so we must use our mind, and reason from cause to effect. If you feel all wrought up, and everything seems to go wrong, perhaps it is because you are suffering the consequences of eating a great variety of food. *(Manuscript Files, 1908)*

115

The digestive organs have an important part to act in our life happiness. God has given us intelligence, that we may learn what we should use as food. Shall we not, as sensible men and women, study whether the things we eat will be in agreement, or whether they will cause trouble? *(Manuscript Files, 1908)*

116

Those who digress occasionally to gratify the taste in eating a fattened turkey or other flesh meats, pervert their appetites, and are not the ones to judge the benefits of the system of health reform. They are controlled by taste, not by principle. *(Testimonies, Volume 2, 1870)*

117

Puddings, custards, sweet cake, and vegetables, all served at the same meal, will cause a disturbance in the stomach. *(1900 Letter)*

"Vegetarian diets have been successful in arresting coronary artery disease."

American Journal of Epidemiology, 1995; 142

118

Some use milk and a large amount of sugar on mush, thinking that they are carrying out health reform. But the sugar and the milk combined are liable to cause fermentation in the stomach, and are thus harmful. *(Christian Temperance and Bible Hygiene, 1890)*

119

The less that condiments and desserts are placed upon our tables, the better it will be for all who partake of the food. All mixed and complicated foods are injurious to the health of human beings. *(1896 Letter)*

120

Many persons bring disease upon themselves by their self-indulgence. They have not lived in accordance with natural law or the principles of strict purity. Others have disregarded the laws of health in their habits of eating and drinking, dressing, or working. *(Ministry of Healing, 1905)*

"Breast cancer rates are lower in populations that consume plant based diets."

American Cancer Society, *Cancer Facts and Figures*, 1994

121

With the majority, their principal anxiety is, What shall I eat? what shall I drink? and wherewith shall I be clothed? Notwithstanding all that is said and written in regard to how we should treat our bodies, appetite is the great law which governs men and women generally. The moral powers are weakened, because men and women will not live in obedience to the laws of health, and make this great subject a personal duty. Parents bequeath to their offspring their own perverted habits, and loathsome diseases corrupt the blood and enervate the brain. The majority of men and women remain in ignorance of the laws of their being, and indulge appetite and passion at the expense of intellect and morals. *(Testimonies, Volume 3, 1872)*

122

You should understand that every organ of the body is to be treated with respect. In the matter of diet, you must reason from cause to effect. *(1908 Letter)*

123

Against every transgression of the laws of life, nature will utter her protest. She bears abuse as long as she can; but finally the retribution comes, and it falls upon the mental as well as the physical powers. Nor does it end with the transgressor; the effects of his indulgence are seen in his offspring, and thus the evil is passed down from generation to generation. The youth of today are a sure index to the future of society; and as we view them, what can we hope for that future? *(How to Live, Book 3, 1866)*

124

The human family have brought upon themselves diseases of various forms by their own wrong habits. They have not studied how to live healthfully, and their transgression of the laws of their being has produced a deplorable state of things. The people have seldom accredited their sufferings to the true cause—their own wrong course of action. They have indulged in intemperance in eating, and made a God of their appetite. In all their habits they have manifested a recklessness in regard to health and life; and when, as the result, sickness has come upon them they have made themselves believe that God was the author of it, when their own wrong course of action has brought the sure result. *(Ministry of Healing, 1905)*

"A vegetarian diet does reduce the occurrence of diabetes."

American Journal of Public Health, 75: 507–512, 1985

125

$\mathcal{D}$isease never comes without a cause. The way is prepared, and disease invited, by disregard of the laws of health. Many suffer in consequence of the transgression of their parents. While they are not responsible for what their parents have done, it is nevertheless their duty to ascertain what are and what are not violations of the laws of health. They should avoid the wrong habits of their parents, and by correct living, place themselves in better conditions. The greater number, however, suffer because of their own wrong course of action. *(Christian Temperance and Bible Hygiene, 1890)*

126

$\mathcal{T}$here is no treatment which can relieve you of your present difficulties while you eat and drink as you do. You can do that for yourselves which the most experienced physician can never do. Regulate your diet. In order to gratify the taste, you frequently place a severe tax upon your digestive organs by receiving into the stomach food which is not the most healthful, and at times in immoderate quantities. This wearies the stomach, and unfits it for the reception of even the most healthful foods. You keep your stomachs constantly debilitated, because of your wrong habits of eating. Your food is made too rich. It is not prepared in a simple, natural manner, but is totally unfitted for the stomach when you have prepared it to suit your taste. *(Testimonies, Volume 6, 1900)*

127

Of all the families I am acquainted with, none need the benefit of the health reform more than yours. You groan under pains and prostrations which you cannot account for, and you try to submit with as good a grace as you can, thinking affliction is your lot, and Providence has thus ordained it. If you could have your eyes opened, and could see the steps taken in your lifetime to walk right into your present condition of poor health, you would be astonished at your blindness in not seeing the real state of the case before. You have created unnatural appetites, and do not derive half that enjoyment from your food which you would if you had not used your appetites wrongfully. You have perverted nature, and have been suffering the consequences, and painful has it been. Nature bears abuse as long as she can without resisting; then she arouses and makes a mighty effort to rid herself of the encumbrances and evil treatment she has suffered. Then come headache, chills, fevers, nervousness, paralysis, and other evils too numerous to mention. A wrong course of eating or drinking destroys health and with it the sweetness of life. Oh, how many times have you purchased what you called a good meal at the expense of a fevered system, loss of appetite, and loss of sleep! Inability to enjoy food, a sleepless night, hours of suffering,—all for a meal in which taste was gratified!
(Testimonies, Volume 2, 1868)

"Scientists at the Royal Perth Hospital in Australia found that people with high blood pressure could indeed reduce it, on a vegetarian diet. They wrote; 'If the usual aim of treatment of mild hypertensives is to reduce systolic blood pressure to below 140mmHg then 30 per cent of those eating a meat-free diet achieved this criteria compared with only 8 per cent on their usual diet."

Clinical and Experimental Pharmacology and Physiology, 1985, 12, pp263–6

128

The mind does not wear out nor break down so often on account of diligent employment and hard study, as on account of eating improper food at improper times, and of careless inattention to the laws of health. Diligent study is not the principal cause of the breaking down of the mental powers. The main cause is improper diet, irregular meals, and a lack of physical exercise. Irregular hours for eating and sleeping sap the brain forces. *(Youth's Instructor, May 31, 1894)*

129

I saw your condition of health, and the ailments you have suffered under so long. I was shown that you have not lived healthfully. Your appetites have been unhealthy, and you have gratified the taste at the expense of the stomach. You have taken into your stomachs articles which it is impossible to convert into good blood. This has laid a heavy tax on the liver, for the reason that the digestive organs are deranged. You both have diseased livers. The health reform would be a great benefit to you both, if you would strictly carry it out. This you have failed to do. Your appetites are morbid, and because you do not relish a plain, simple diet, composed of unbolted wheat flour, vegetables and fruits prepared without spices or grease, you are continually transgressing the laws which God has established in your system. While you do this, you must suffer the penalty; for to every transgression is affixed a penalty. Yet you wonder at your continued poor health. Be assured that God will not work a miracle to save you from the result of your own course of action. *(Testimonies, Volume 2, 1868)*

130

The stomach may never entirely recover health after long abuse; but a proper course of diet will save further debility, and many will recover more or less fully. It is not easy to prescribe rules that will meet every case; but with attention to right principles in eating, great reforms may be made, and the cook need not be continually toiling to tempt the appetite. *(Ministry of Healing, 1905)*

131

Those foods should be chosen that best supply the elements needed for building up the body. In this choice, appetite is not a safe guide. Through wrong habits of eating, the appetite has become perverted. Often it demands food that impairs health and causes weakness instead of strength. We cannot safely be guided by the customs of society. The disease and suffering that everywhere prevail are largely due to popular errors in regard to diet. *(Ministry of Healing, 1905)*

"A diet that is high in animal protein- as opposed to vegetable proteins-particularly increases the excretion of calcium."
Journal of Clinical Endocrinological Metabolism, Jan 1988, 66 (1), pp140–6

132

Many are suffering, and many are going into the grave, because of the indulgence of appetite. They eat what suits their perverted taste, thus weakening the digestive organs and injuring their power to assimilate the food that is to sustain life. This brings on acute disease, and too often death follows. *(Testimonies, Volume 2, 1868)*

133

$\mathcal{L}$et us never bear testimony against health reform by failing to use wholesome, palatable food in place of the harmful articles of diet that we have discarded. *(1902 Letter)*

134

$\mathcal{T}$hose who, after seeing their mistakes, have courage to change their habits, will find that the reformatory process requires a struggle and much perseverance; but when correct tastes are once formed, they will realize that the use of the food which they formerly regarded as harmless, was slowly but surely laying the foundation for dyspepsia and other diseases. *(Testimonies, Volume 9, 1909)*

135

$\mathcal{M}$any spoil their dispositions by eating improperly. We should be just as careful to learn the lessons of health reform as we are to have our studies perfectly prepared; for the habits that we adopt in this direction are helping to form our characters for the future life. It is possible for one to spoil his spiritual experience by an ill-use of the stomach. *(1908 Letter)*

136

$\mathcal{O}$vertaxing the stomach is a common sin, and when too much food is used, the entire system is burdened. Life and vitality, instead of being increased, are decreased. This is as Satan plans to have it. Man uses up his vital forces in unnecessary labor in taking care of an excess of food. *(1895 Letter)*

> "Since the 1920s scientists have known that diets that are high in protein cause calcium to be lost through the urine."
>
> *Journal of Nutrition,* 1981, 111, pp 552–3

137

*I*ndulgence of appetite is the greatest cause of physical and mental debility, and lies largely at the foundation of feebleness and premature death. *(Testimonies, Volume 9, 1909)*

138

*N*early all the members of the human family eat more than the system requires. This excess decays and becomes a putrid mass . . . If more food, even of a simple quality, is placed in the stomach than the living machinery requires, this surplus becomes a burden. The system makes desperate efforts to dispose of it, and this extra work causes a tired, weary feeling. Some who are continually eating call this all-gone feeling hunger, but it is caused by the overworked condition of the digestive organs. *(1896 Letter)*

139

*I*t is possible to eat immoderately, even of wholesome food. It does not follow that because one has discarded the use of hurtful articles of diet, he can eat just as much as he pleases. Overeating, no matter what the quality of the food, clogs the living machine, and thus hinders it in its work. *(Christian Temperance and Bible Hygiene, 1890)*

140

By taking too much food, we not only improvidently waste the blessings of God, provided for the necessities of nature, but do great injury to the whole system. We defile the temple of God; it is weakened and crippled; and nature cannot do its work wisely and well, as God has made provision that it should. Because of the selfish indulgence of his appetite, man has oppressed nature's power by compelling it to do work it should never be required to do. Were all men acquainted with the living, human machinery, they would not be guilty of doing this, unless, indeed, they loved self-indulgence so well that they would continue their suicidal course and die a premature death, or live for years a burden to themselves and to their friends. *(1895 Letter)*

141

Intemperance in eating, even of healthful food, will have an injurious effect upon the system, and will blunt the mental and moral faculties. *(Signs, September 1, 1887)*

"Diets low in saturated fats, high in omega-3 fatty acids and high in fruits, vegetables, nuts, and whole grains are the best for your heart."

Journal of the American Medical Association, Nov. 27, 2002

142

Gluttonous feasts, and food taken into the stomach at untimely seasons, leave an influence upon every fiber of the system; and the mind also is seriously affected by what we eat and drink. *(Health Reform, June, 1878)*

143

$\mathcal{C}$ustom has decreed that the food should be placed upon the tables in courses. Not knowing what is coming next, one may eat a sufficiency of food which perhaps is not the best suited to him. When the last course is brought on, he often ventures to overstep the bounds, and take the tempting dessert, which, however, proves anything but good for him. If all the food intended for a meal is placed on the table at the beginning, one has opportunity to make the best choice. *(Ministry of Healing, 1905)*

144

$\mathcal{T}$he surplus food burdens the system, and produces morbid, feverish conditions. It calls an undue amount of blood to the stomach, causing the limbs and extremities to chill quickly. It lays a heavy tax on the digestive organs, and when these organs have accomplished their task, there is a feeling of faintness or languor. Some who are continually overeating call this all-gone feeling hunger; but it is caused by the overworked condition of the digestive organs. At times there is numbness of the brain, with disinclination to mental or physical effort. These unpleasant symptoms are felt because nature has accomplished her work at an unnecessary outlay of vital force, and is thoroughly exhausted. The stomach is saying, "Give me rest." But with many the faintness is interpreted as a demand for more food; so instead of giving the stomach rest, another burden it placed upon it. As a consequence the digestive organs are often worn out when they should be capable of doing good work. *(Ministry of Healing, 1905)*

"High fruit and vegetable intake reduces stroke risk."
Journal of the American Medical Association, 282:1233–39, Oct. 5, 1999

145

Some do not exercise control over their appetites, but indulge taste at the expense of health. As the result, the brain is clouded, their thoughts are sluggish, and they fail to accomplish what they might if they were self-denying and abstemious. *(Testimonies, Volume 4, 1880)*

146

Many who discard flesh meats and other gross and injurious articles think that because their food is simple and wholesome they may indulge appetite without restraint, and they eat to excess, sometimes to gluttony. This is an error. The digestive organs should not be burdened with a quantity or quality of food which it will tax the system to appropriate. *(Ministry of Healing, 1905)*

147

As a people, with all our profession of health reform, we eat too much. *(Christian Temperance and Hygiene Healing, 1890)*

148

Many who have adopted the health reform have left off everything hurtful; but does it follow that because they have left off these things, they can eat just as much as they please? They sit down to the table, and instead of considering how much they should eat, they give themselves up to appetite and eat to great excess. And the stomach has all it can do, or all it should do, the rest of that day, to worry away with the burden imposed upon it. *(Testimonies, Volume 2, 1870)*

149

A clogged stomach means a clogged brain. *(Ministry of Healing, 1905)*

150

*T*he Lord has instructed me that as a general rule, we place too much food in the stomach. Many make themselves uncomfortable by overeating, and sickness is often the result. The Lord did not bring this punishment on them. They brought it on themselves; and God desires them to realize that pain is the result of transgression. *(Manuscript Files, 1901)*

"Women eating the highest amounts of red meats, sweets, french fries and refined grains had 1.5 times the risk of colon cancer of women who ate more fruits, vegetables, fish and whole grains."
Archives of Internal Medicine, Volume 4, Number 36; February 14, 2003

151

*M*any writers and speakers fail here. After eating heartily they give themselves to sedentary occupations, reading, study, or writing, allowing no time for physical exercise. As a consequence, the free flow of thought and words is checked. They cannot write or speak with the force and intensity necessary in order to reach the heart; their efforts are tame and fruitless. Those upon whom rest important responsibilities, those, above all, who are guardians of spiritual interests, should be men of keen feeling and quick perception. More than others, they need to be temperate in eating. Rich and luxurious food should have no place upon their tables. *(Ministry of Healing, 1905)*

152

Frequently you place in your stomach double the quantity of food your system requires. This food decays; your breath becomes offensive; your catarrhal difficulties are aggravated; your stomach is overworked; and life and energy are called from the brain to work the mill which grinds the material you have placed in your stomach. In this, you have shown little mercy to yourself. *(1895 Letter)*

153

You are a gourmand when at the table. This is one great cause of your forgetfulness and loss of memory. You say things which I know you have said, and then turn square about, and say that you said something entirely different. I knew this, but passed it over as the sure result of overeating. Of what use would it be to speak about it? It would not cure the evil. *(1895 Letter)*

154

The reason why many of our ministers complain of sickness is, they fail to take sufficient exercise, and indulge in overeating. They do not realize that such a course endangers the strongest constitution. Those who, like yourself, are sluggish in temperament, should eat very sparingly, and not shun physical taxation. Many of our ministers are digging their graves with their teeth. The system, in taking care of the burden placed upon the digestive organs, suffers, and a severe draft is made upon the brain. For every offense committed against the laws of health, the transgressor must pay the penalty in his own body. *(Testimonies, Volume 4, 1880)*

155

Overeating is especially harmful to those who are sluggish in temperament; these should eat sparingly, and take plenty of physical exercise. There are men and women of excellent natural ability who do not accomplish half what they might if they would exercise self-control in the denial of appetite. *(Ministry of Healing, 1905)*

"When I was 88 years old, I gave up meat entirely and switched to a plant-foods diet following a slight stroke. During the following months, I not only lost 50 pounds but gained strength in my legs and picked up stamina. Now, at age 93, I'm on the same plant-based diet, and I still don't eat any meat or dairy products. I either swim, walk, or paddle a canoe daily and I feel the best I've felt since my heart problems began."

Dr. Benjamin Spock, Nutrition Advocate, 1996

156

Crime and disease have increased with every succeeding generation. Intemperance in eating and drinking, and the indulgence of the baser passions, have benumbed the nobler faculties of man. Reason, instead of being the ruler, has come to be the slave of appetite to an alarming extent. An increasing desire for rich food has been indulged, until it has become the fashion to crowd all the delicacies possible into the stomach. Especially at parties of pleasure is the appetite indulged with but little restraint. Rich dinners and late suppers are served, consisting of highly seasoned meats, with rich sauces, cakes, pies, ices, tea, coffee, etc. No wonder that, with such a diet, people have sallow complexions, and suffer untold agonies from dyspepsia. *(Testimonies, Volume 2, 1868)*

157

Sometimes the result of overeating is felt at once. In other cases there is no sensation of pain; but the digestive organs lose their vital force, and the foundation of physical strength is undermined. *(Ministry of Healing, 1905)*

158

At bountiful tables, men often eat much more than can be easily digested. The overburdened stomach cannot do its work properly. The result is a disagreeable feeling of dullness in the brain, and the mind does not act quickly. *(Testimonies, Volume 7, 1902)*

159

There is a class who profess to believe the truth, who do not use tobacco, snuff, tea, or coffee, yet they are guilty of gratifying the appetite in a different manner. They crave highly seasoned meats, with rich gravies, and their appetite has become so perverted that they cannot be satisfied with even meat, unless prepared in a manner most injurious. The stomach is fevered, the digestive organs are taxed, and yet the stomach labors hard to dispose of the load forced upon it. After the stomach has performed its task it becomes exhausted, which causes faintness. Here many are deceived, and think that it is the want of food which produces such feelings, and without giving the stomach time to rest, they take more food, which for the time removes the faintness. And the more the appetite is indulged, the more will be its clamors for gratification. This faintness is generally the result of meat eating, and eating frequently, and too much. *(Spiritual Gifts, Book 4, 1864)*

> "A high ratio of dietary animal to vegetable protein increases the rate of bone loss and the risk of fracture in postmenopausal women."
> *American Journal of Clinical Nutrition*, 2001 Jan; 73(1):118–22

160

*M*any eat three times a day, and again just before going to bed. In a short time the digestive organs are worn out, for they have had no time to rest. These become miserable dyspeptics, and wonder what has made them so. The cause has brought the sure result. *(Spiritual Gifts, Book 4, 1864)*

161

*C*arefully consider your diet. Study from cause to effect. Cultivate self-control. Keep appetite under the control of reason. Never abuse the stomach by overeating, but do not deprive yourself of the wholesome, palatable food that health demands. *(Ministry of Healing, 1905)*

162

*T*he stomach is not fevered with meat, and overtaxed, but is in a healthy condition, and can readily perform its task. There should be no delay in reform. Efforts should be made to preserve carefully the remaining strength of the vital forces, by lifting off every overtaxing burden. The stomach may never fully recover health, but a proper course of diet will save further debility, and many will recover more or less, unless they have gone very far in gluttonous self-murder. *(Spiritual Gifts, Book 4, 1864)*

163

*I*f they cannot at first enjoy plain food, they should fast until they can. That fast will prove to them of greater benefit than medicine, for the abused stomach will find that rest which it has long needed, and real hunger can be satisfied with a plain diet. It will take time for the taste to recover from the abuses which it has received, and to gain its natural tone. But perseverance in a self-denying course of eating and drinking will soon make plain, wholesome food palatable, and it will soon be eaten with greater satisfaction than the epicure enjoys over his rich dainties. *(Spiritual Gifts, Book 4, 1864)*

164

*M*any are incapacitated for both mentally and physically by overeating and the gratification of the lustful passions. The animal propensities are strengthened, while the moral and spiritual nature is enfeebled. *(Review and Herald, January 25, 1881)*

"An association was found between consumption of red meat, particularly processed meat, and risk of colorectal cancer, which corresponds with current advice to limit intakes of red meat and meat products."

Cancer Epidemiology, Biomarkers and Prevention, 2001; 10: 439–446

165

*M*uch tact and discretion should be employed in preparing nourishing food to take the place of that which has constituted the diet of many families. This effort requires faith in God, earnestness of purpose, and a willingness to help one another. *(1902 Letter)*

166

To deny appetite requires decision of character. For want of this decision multitudes are ruined. Weak, pliable, easily led, many men and women fail utterly of becoming what God desires them to be. Those who are destitute of decision of character cannot make a success of the daily work of overcoming. The world is full of besotted, intemperate, weak-minded men and women, and how hard it is for them to become genuine Christians. *(1903 Letter)*

167

Many students are deplorably ignorant of the fact that diet exerts a powerful influence upon the health. Some have never made a determined effort to control the appetite, or to observe proper rules in regard to diet. They eat too much, even at their meals, and some eat between meals whenever the temptation is presented. *(Christian Temperance and Bible Hygiene, 1890)*

168

Many are enfeebling their digestive organs by indulging perverted appetite. The power of the human constitution to resist the abuses put upon it is wonderful; but persistent wrong habits in excessive eating and drinking will enfeeble every function of the body. Let these feeble ones consider what they might have been, had they lived temperately, and promoted health instead of abusing it. In the gratification of perverted appetite and passion, even professed Christians cripple nature in her work and lessen physical, mental, and moral power. Some who are doing this, claim to be sanctified to God; but such a claim is without foundation. *(Testimonies, Volume 5, 1882)*

169

A second meal should never be eaten until the stomach has had time to rest from the labor of digesting the preceding meal. If a third meal be eaten at all, it should be light, and several hours before going to bed. But with many, the poor, tired stomach may complain of weariness in vain. More food is forced upon it, which sets the digestive organs in motion, again to perform the same round of labor through the sleeping hours. The sleep of such is generally disturbed with unpleasant dreams, and in the morning they awake un-refreshed. *(Spiritual Gifts, Book 4, 1864)*

"Vegetarian diets low in fat or saturated fat have been used successfully as part of comprehensive health programs to reverse severe coronary artery disease."

Journal of the American Medical Association, 1995; 274

170

*M*any indulge in the pernicious habit of eating just before sleeping hours. They may have taken three regular meals; yet because they feel a sense of faintness, as though hungry, will eat a lunch or fourth meal. By indulging this wrong practice, it has become a habit, and they feel as though they could not sleep without taking a lunch before retiring. In many cases, the cause of this faintness is because the digestive organs have been already too severely taxed through the day in disposing of unwholesome food forced upon the stomach too frequently, and in too great quantities. The digestive organs thus taxed become weary, and need a period of entire rest from labor to recover their exhausted energies. *(How to Live, Book 1, 1865)*

171

Thousands who might have lived, have passed into the grave, physical, mental, and moral wrecks, because they sacrificed all their powers to the indulgence of appetite. The necessity for the men of this generation to call to their aid the power of the will, strengthened by the grace of God, in order to withstand the temptations of Satan, and resist the least indulgence of perverted appetite, is far greater than it was several generations ago. But the present generation have less power of self-control than had those who lived then. *(Christian Temperance and Bible Hygiene, 1890)*

172

Few have moral stamina to resist temptation, especially of the appetite, and to practice self-denial. To some it is a temptation too strong to be resisted to see others eat the third meal; and they imagine they are hungry, when the feeling is not a call of the stomach for food, but a desire of the mind that has not been fortified with firm principle, and disciplined to self-denial. The walls of self-control and self-restriction should not in a single instance be weakened and broken down. *(Testimonies, Volume 4, 1881)*

173

It is the custom and order of society to take a slight breakfast. But this is not the best way to treat the stomach. At breakfast time the stomach is in a better condition to take care of more food than at the second or third meal of the day. The habit of eating a sparing breakfast and a large dinner is wrong. Make your breakfast correspond more nearly to the heartiest meal of the day. *(1884 Letter)*

> "Plant sources of protein alone can provide adequate amounts of essential amino acids if a variety of plant foods are consumed and energy needs are met. Research suggests that complementary proteins do not need to be consumed at the same time and that consumption of various sources of amino acids over the course of the day should ensure adequate nitrogen retention and use in healthy persons."
>
> *Journal of the American Dietetic Association,* November 1997, 97(1) citing the *American Journal of Clinical Nutrition,* 1994; 59 (suppl 5):1203–1212

174

I am given a message to give to you: Eat at regular periods. By wrong habits of eating, you are preparing yourself for future suffering. It is not always safe to comply with invitations to meals, even though given by your brethren and friends, who wish to lavish upon you many kinds of food. You know that you can eat two or three kinds of food at a meal without injury to your digestive organs. When you are invited out to a meal, shun the many varieties of food that those who have invited you set before you. This you must do if you would be a faithful sentinel. When food is placed before us, which, if eaten, would cause the digestive organs hours of hard work, we must not, if we eat this food, blame those who set it before us for the result. *(1905 Letter)*

175

In most cases, two meals a day are preferable to three. Supper, when taken at an early hour, interferes with the digestion of the previous meal. When taken later, it is not itself digested before bedtime. Thus the stomach fails of securing proper rest. The sleep is disturbed, the brain and nerves are wearied, the appetite for breakfast is impaired, the whole system is un-refreshed, and is unready for the day's duties. *(Education, 1903)*

175

Regularity in eating should be carefully observed. Nothing should be eaten between meals, no confectionery, nuts, fruits, or food of any kind. Irregularities in eating destroy the healthful tone of the digestive organs, to the detriment of health and cheerfulness. And when the children come to the table, they do not relish wholesome food; their appetites crave that which is hurtful for them. *(Ministry of Healing, 1905)*

"Swedish researchers who enrolled 66 arthritis patients in a one-year study assigned 38 to a gluten-free, vegan diet and 28 to a non-vegan diet (control group). Forty percent of people in the vegan group improved compared to just one person in the control group."

Rheumatology, 2001; 40:1175–9

177

Neither should the meals be delayed one or two hours, to suit circumstances, or in order that a certain amount of work may be accomplished. The stomach calls for food at the time it is accustomed to receive it. If that time is delayed, the vitality of the system decreases, and finally reaches so low an ebb that the appetite is entirely gone. If food is then taken, the stomach is unable to properly care for it. The food cannot be converted into good blood. *(Manuscript Files, 1876)*

178

The stomach may be so educated as to desire food eight times a day, and feel faint if it is not supplied. But this is no argument in favor of so frequent eating. *(Review and Herald, May 8, 1883)*

179

*M*any turn from light and knowledge, and sacrifice principle to taste. They eat when the system needs no food, and at irregular intervals, because they have no moral stamina to resist inclination. As the result, the abused stomach rebels, and suffering follows. Regularity in eating is very important for health of body and serenity of mind. Never should a morsel of food pass the lips between meals. *(Christian Temperance and Bible Hygiene, 1890)*

180

*F*or persons of sedentary habits, late suppers are particularly harmful. With them the disturbance created is often the beginning of disease that ends in death. In many cases the faintness that leads to a desire for food is felt because the digestive organs have been too severely taxed during the day. After disposing of one meal, the digestive organs need rest. At least five or six hours should intervene between the meals; and most persons who give the plan a trial, will find that two meals a day are better than three. *(Ministry of Healing, 1905)*

181

*A*fter the regular meal is eaten, the stomach should be allowed to rest for five hours. Not a particle of food should be introduced into the stomach till the next meal. In this interval the stomach will perform its work, and will then be in a condition to receive more food. In no case should the meals be irregular. If dinner is eaten an hour or two before the usual time, the stomach is unprepared for the new burden; for it has not yet disposed of the food eaten at the previous meal, and has not vital force for new work. Thus the system is overtaxed. *(Manuscript Files, 1876)*

182

The stomach must have careful attention. It must not be kept in continual operation. Give this misused and much-abused organ some peace and quiet and rest. After the stomach has done its work for one meal, do not crowd more work upon it before it has had a chance to rest and before a sufficient supply of gastric juice is provided by nature to care for more food. Five hours at least should elapse between each meal, and always bear in mind that if you would give it a trial, you would find that two meals are better than three. *(1896 Letter)*

"One study tested a mostly raw vegan diet in 30 patients with fibromyalgia, a syndrome of chronic fatigue, pain, poor sleep, depression, and anxiety. After several months on the diet, 19 participants showed signs of improvement in range of motion, flexibility, and other measures."

BMC Complementary Alternative Medicine, 2001; 1:7

183

Regularity in eating is of vital importance. There should be a specified time for each meal. At this time, let every one eat what the system requires, and then take nothing more until the next meal. There are many who eat when the system needs no food, at irregular intervals, and between meals, because they have not sufficient strength of will to resist inclination. When traveling, some are constantly nibbling if anything eatable is within their reach. This is very injurious. If travelers would eat regularly of food that is simple and nutritious, they would not feel so great weariness, nor suffer so much from sickness. *(Ministry of Healing, 1905)*

"Ten healthy participants were asked to follow an Atkins-style, carbohydrate-restricted diet for two weeks and then follow a moderately carbohydrate-restricted diet for four more weeks under close monitoring. It turned out that the meaty diets increased their calcium loss by 55 percent. Researchers concluded that a high-protein diet presents a marked acid load to the kidneys, increase the risk for kidney stones, and may increase the risk for bone loss."

American Journal of Kidney Disease, 2002; 2:265–74

184

Children are generally untaught in regard to the importance of when, how, and what they should eat. They are permitted to indulge their tastes freely, to eat at all hours, to help themselves to fruit when it tempts their eyes, and this, with the pie, cake, bread and butter, and sweetmeats eaten almost constantly, makes them gourmands and dyspeptics. The digestive organs, like a mill which is continually kept running, become enfeebled, vital force is called from the brain to aid the stomach in its overwork, and thus the mental powers are weakened. The unnatural stimulation and wear of the vital forces make them nervous, impatient of restraint, self-willed, and irritable. *(Health Reformer, May, 1877)*

185

When traveling, some are almost constantly nibbling, if there is anything within their reach. This is a most pernicious practice. Animals that do not have reason, and that know nothing of mental taxation, may do this without injury, but they are no criterion for rational beings, who have mental powers that should be used for God and humanity. *(Health Reformer, June, 1878)*

186

*I*t is quite a common custom with people of the world to eat three times a day, beside eating at irregular intervals between meals; and the last meal is generally the most hearty, and is often taken just before retiring. This is reversing the natural order; a hearty meal should never be taken so late in the day. Should these persons change their practice, and eat but two meals a day, and nothing between meals, not even an apple, a nut, or any kind of fruit, the result would be seen in a good appetite and greatly improved health. *(Review and Herald, July 29, 1884)*

187

A poor quality of food, cooked in an improper manner, and insufficient in quantity, cannot make good blood. Flesh meats and rich food, and an impoverished diet, will produce the same results. *(Testimonies, Volume 2, 1870)*

"Studies indicate that vegetarians often have lower morbidity and mortality rates from several chronic degenerative diseases than do non-vegetarians. Although non-dietary factors, including physical activity and abstinence from smoking and alcohol, may play a role, diet is clearly a contributing factor."

British Medical Journal, 1996; 313:775–779.

188

*M*any eat at all hours, regardless of the laws of health. Then gloom covers the mind. How can men be honored with divine enlightenment, when they are so reckless in their habits, so inattentive to the light which God has given in regard to these things? *(Gospel Workers, 1892)*

189

*I*ntemperate eating is often the cause of sickness, and what nature most needs is to be relieved of the undue burden that has been placed upon her. In many cases of sickness, the very best remedy is for the patient to fast for a meal or two, that the overworked organs of digestion may have an opportunity to rest. *(Ministry of Healing, 1905)*

190

*O*vereating, even of the simplest food, benumbs the sensitive nerves of the brain, and weakens its vitality. *(Testimonies, Volume 2, 1870)*

191

*I*n cases of severe fever, abstinence from food for a short time will lessen the fever, and make the use of water more effectual. But the acting physician needs to understand the real condition of the patient, and not allow him to be restricted in diet for a great length of time until his system becomes enfeebled. While the fever is raging, food may irritate and excite the blood; but as soon as the strength of the fever is broken, nourishment should be given in a careful, judicious manner. If food is withheld too long, the stomach's craving for it will create fever, which will be relieved by a proper allowance of food of a right quality. It gives nature something to work upon. If there is a great desire expressed for food, even during the fever, to gratify that desire with a moderate amount of simple food would be less injurious than for the patient to be denied. When he can get his mind upon nothing else, nature will not be overburdened with a small portion of simple food. *(Christian Temperance and Bible Hygiene, 1890)*

192

*I*ndulging in eating too frequently, and in too large quantities, overtaxes the digestive organs, and produces a feverish state of the system. The blood becomes impure, and then diseases of various kinds occur. The sufferers in such cases can do for themselves that which others cannot do as well for them. They should commence to relieve nature of the load they have forced upon her. They should remove the cause. Fast a short time, and give the stomach a chance for rest. Reduce the feverish state of the system by a careful and understanding application of water. These efforts will help nature in her struggles to free the system of impurities. *(Spiritual Gifts, Book 4, 1864)*

> "This study showed that patients with moderate-to-severe rheumatoid arthritis (RA), who switch to a low-fat, vegan diet can experience significant reductions in RA symptoms."
>
> *Journal of Alternative and Complementary Medicine,* February, 2002, 8; 1

193

*N*arrow ideas, and overstraining of small points, have been a great injury to the cause of hygiene. There may be such an effort at economy in the preparation of food, that, instead of a healthful diet, it becomes a poverty-stricken diet. What is the result?—Poverty of the blood. I have seen several cases of disease most difficult to cure, which were due to impoverished diet. The persons thus afflicted were not compelled by poverty to adopt a meager diet, but did so in order to follow out their own erroneous ideas of what constitutes health reform. Day after day, meal after meal, the same articles of food were prepared without variation, until dyspepsia and general debility resulted. *(Testimonies, Volume 2, 1870)*

194

*M*en need to think less about what they shall eat and drink of temporal food, and much more in regard to the food from heaven, that will give tone and vitality to the whole religious experience. *(1896 Letter)*

"U.S. children who are overweight or obese: 25%"
Archives of Pediatric and Adolescent Medicine, 1995; 149:1085–91

"U.S. children who eat the recommended levels of fruits, vegetables, and grains: 1%"
Pediatrics, Sept 1997, pp 323–29

195

*T*here are some who would be benefited more by abstinence from food for a day or two every week than by any amount of treatment or medical advice. To fast one day a week would be of incalculable benefit to them. *(Testimonies, Volume 7, 1902)*

196

*W*e advise you to change your habits of living; but while you do this we caution you to move understandingly. I am acquainted with families who have changed from a meat diet to one that is impoverished. Their food is so poorly prepared that the stomach loathes it, and such have told me that the health reform did not agree with them; that they were decreasing in physical strength. Here is one reason why some have not been successful in their efforts to simplify their food. They have a poverty-stricken diet. Food is prepared without painstaking, and there is a continual sameness. *(1901 Letter)*

197

*I*n order to keep pace with fashion, nature has been abused, instead of being consulted. Mothers sometimes depend upon a hireling, or a nursing bottle must be substituted, for the maternal breast. And one of the most delicate and gratifying duties a mother can perform for her dependent offspring, which blends her life with its own, and which awakens the most holy feelings in the hearts of women, is sacrificed to fashion's murderous folly. There are mothers who will sacrifice their maternal duties in nursing their children simply because it is too much trouble to be confined to their offspring, which is the fruit of their own body. *(Testimonies, Volume 6, 1900)*

198

*S*ome have limited themselves to a diet that cannot sustain them in health. They have not provided nourishing food to take the place of injurious articles; and they have not considered that tact and ingenuity must be exercised in preparing food in the most healthful manner. The system must be properly nourished in order to perform its work. It is contrary to health reform, after cutting off the great variety of unwholesome dishes, to go to the opposite extreme, reducing the quantity and quality of the food to a low standard. Instead of health reform this is health deform. *(1886 Letter)*

199

I have been shown that many take a wrong view of the health reform, and adopt too poor a diet. They subsist upon a cheap, poor quality of food, prepared without care or reference to the nourishment of the system. *(Testimonies, Volume 2, 1870)*

200

The time will come when we may have to discard some of the articles of diet we now use, such as milk and cream and eggs; but my message is that you must not bring yourself to a time of trouble beforehand, and thus afflict yourself with death. Wait till the Lord prepares the way before you. But I wish to say that when the time comes that it is no longer safe to use milk, cream, butter, and eggs, God will reveal this. *(Testimonies, Volume 2, 1868)*

201

Many are debilitated from disease, and need nourishing, well-cooked food. Health reformers, above all others, should be careful to avoid extremes. The body must have sufficient nourishment. *(Christian Temperance and Bible Hygiene, 1890)*

202

The importance of training children to right dietetic habits can hardly be overestimated. The little ones need to learn that they eat to live, not live to eat. The training should begin with the infant in its mother's arms. The child should be given food only at regular intervals, and less frequently as it grows older. It should not be given sweets, or the food of older persons, which it is unable to digest. Care and regularity in the feeding of infants will not only promote health, and thus tend to make them quiet and sweet-tempered, but will lay the foundation of habits and will be a blessing to them in after years. *(Ministry of Healing, 1905)*

"Osteoporosis is caused by a number of things, one of the most important being too much dietary protein."

Science, 1986; 233(4763)

"40% of the world's cancer cases could be prevented through the adoption of diets rich in grains, fruit and vegetables."

American Institute for Cancer Research; World Cancer Fund 10/16/97

203

The best food for the infant is the food that nature provides. Of this it should not be needlessly deprived. It is a heartless thing for a mother, for the sake of convenience or social enjoyment, to seek to free herself from the tender office of nursing her little one. The mother who permits her child to be nourished by another should consider well what the result may be. To a greater or less degree the nurse imparts her own temper and temperament to the nursing child. *(Signs, September 13, 1910)*

204

You need not go into the water, or into the fire, but take the middle path, avoiding all extremes. Do not let it appear that you are one-sided, ill-balanced managers. Do not have a meager, poor diet. Do not let any one influence you to have the diet poverty-stricken. Have your food prepared in a healthful, tasteful manner; have your food prepared with a nicety that will correctly represent health reform. The great backsliding upon health reform is because unwise minds have handled it and carried it to such extremes that it has disgusted in place of converting people to it. I have been where these radical ideas have been carried out. Vegetables prepared with only water, and everything else in like manner. This kind of cookery is health deform, and there are some minds so constituted that they will accept anything that bears the features of rigorous diet or reform of any kind. *(Ministry of Healing, 1905)*

205

The period in which the infant receives its nourishment from the mother is critical. Many mothers, while nursing their infants, have been permitted to overlabor, and to heat their blood in cooking, and the nursling has been seriously affected, not only with fevered nourishment from the mother's breast, but its blood has been poisoned by the unhealthy diet of the mother, which has fevered her whole system, thereby affecting the food of the infant. The infant will also be affected by the condition of the mother's mind. If she is unhappy, easily agitated, irritable, giving vent to outbursts of passion, the nourishment the infant receives from its mother will be inflamed, often producing colic, spasms, and, in some instances, causing convulsions and fits. The character also of the child is more or less affected by the nature of the nourishment received from the mother. *(How to Live, Book 2, 1865)*

206

Not all who profess to believe in dietetic reform are really reformers. With many persons the reform consists merely in discarding certain unwholesome foods. *(Ministry of Healing, 1905)*

207

Highly seasoned meats, followed by rich pastry, is wearing out the vital organs of the digestion of children. Were they accustomed to plain, wholesome food, their appetites would not crave unnatural luxuries and mixed preparations. Meat given to children is not the best thing to ensure success. To educate your children to subsist on a meat diet would be harmful to them. It is much easier to create an unnatural appetite than to correct and reform the taste after it has become second nature. *(1896 Letter)*

208

The first education children should receive from the mother in infancy should be in regard to their physical health. They should be allowed only plain food, of that quality that would preserve to them the best condition of health, and that should be partaken of only at regular periods, not oftener than three times a day, and two meals would be better than three. *(How to Live, Book 2, 1865)*

"Lower breast cancer rates have not been observed in Western vegetarians, but cross-cultural data indicate that breast cancer rates are lower in populations that consume plant-based diets."

American Journal of Clinical Nutrition, 1990; 51:798–803

209

Children are also fed too frequently, which produces feverishness and suffering in various ways. The stomach should not be kept constantly at work, but should have its periods of rest. Without it children will be peevish and irritable and frequently sick. *(Health Reformer, September, 1866)*

210

As children emerge from babyhood, great care should still be taken in educating their tastes and appetite. Often they are permitted to eat what they choose and when they choose, without reference to health. The pains and money so often lavished upon unwholesome dainties lead the young to think that the highest object in life, and that which yields the greatest amount of happiness, is to be able to indulge the appetite. The result of this training is gluttony, then comes sickness, which is usually followed by dosing with poisonous drugs. *(Ministry of Healing, 1905)*

211

Your children should not be allowed to eat candies, fruit, nuts, or anything in the line of food, between their meals. Two meals a day are better for them than three. If the parents set the example, and move from principle, the children will soon fall into line. Irregularities in eating destroy the healthy tone of the digestive organs, and when your children come to the table, they do not relish wholesome food; their appetites crave that which is the most hurtful for them. Many times your children have suffered from fever and ague brought on by improper eating, when their parents were accountable for their sickness. It is the duty of parents to see that their children form habits conducive to health, thereby saving much distress. *(Testimonies, Volume 4, 1880)*

"Vegetarian diets low in fat or saturated fat have been used successfully as part of comprehensive health programs to reverse severe coronary artery disease."

Archives of Family Medicine, 1995; 4:551–554.

212

Parents may have transmitted to their children tendencies to appetite and passion, which will make more difficult the work of educating and training these children to be strictly temperate, and to have pure and virtuous habits. If the appetite for unhealthful food and for stimulants and narcotics, has been transmitted to them as a legacy from their parents, what a fearfully solemn responsibility rests upon the parents to counteract the evil tendencies which they have given to their children! How earnestly and diligently should the parents work to do their duty, in faith and hope, to their unfortunate offspring! *(Testimonies, Volume 3, 1875)*

213

$f$ood should be so simple that its preparation will not absorb all the time of the mother. It is true, care should be taken to furnish the table with healthful food prepared in a wholesome and inviting manner. Do not think that anything you can carelessly throw together to serve as food is good enough for the children. But less time should be devoted to the preparation of unhealthful dishes for the table, to please a perverted taste, and more time to the education and training of the children. *(Christian Temperance and Bible Hygiene, 1890)*

214

Gross and stimulating food fevers the blood, excites the nervous system, and too often dulls the moral perceptions, so that reason and conscience are overborne by the sensual impulses. It is difficult, and often well-nigh impossible, for one who is intemperate in diet to exercise patience and self-control. Hence the special importance of allowing children, whose characters are yet uniformed, to have only such food as is healthful and un-stimulating. *(Testimonies, Volume 2, 1868)*

215

$m$any a mother sets a table that is a snare to her family. Flesh meats, butter, cheese, rich pastry, spiced foods, and condiments are freely partaken of by both old and young. These things do their work in deranging the stomach, exciting the nerves, and enfeebling the intellect. The blood-making organs cannot convert such things into good blood. The grease cooked in the food renders it difficult of digestion. *(Christian Temperance and Bible Hygiene, 1890)*

216

*H*abits once formed are hard to overcome. The reform should begin with the mother before the birth of her children; and if God's instructions were faithfully obeyed, intemperance would not exist. *(Health Reformer, September, 1871)*

217

*B*ut even health reformers can err in the quantity of food. They can eat immoderately of a healthful quality of food. Some in this house err in the quality. They have never taken their position upon health reform. They have chosen to eat and drink what they pleased and when they pleased. They are injuring their systems in this way. Not only this, but they are injuring their families by placing upon their tables a feverish diet, which will increase the animal passions of their children, and lead them to care but little for heavenly things. *(Health Reformer, December, 1870)*

218

*P*arents should make it their first object to become intelligent in regard to the proper manner of dealing with their children, that they may secure to them sound minds in sound bodies. The principles of temperance should be carried out in all the details of home life. *(Christian Temperance and Bible Hygiene, 1890)*

219

One little girl was partaking of her boiled ham, and spiced pickles, and bread and butter, when she espied a plate I was eating from. Here was something she did not have, and she refused to eat. The girl of six years said she would have a plate. I thought it was the nice red apple I was eating she desired; and although we had a limited amount, I felt such pity for the parents, that I gave her a fine apple. She snatched it from my hand, and disdainfully threw it quickly to the car floor. I thought, This child, if permitted to thus have her own way, will indeed bring her mother to shame. This exhibition of passion was the result of the mother's course of indulgence. The quality of food she provided for her child was a continual tax to the digestive organs. *(Health Reformer, December, 1870)*

220

I noticed a boy of three years, who was suffering with diarrhea. He had quite a fever, but seemed to think all he needed was food. He was calling, every few minutes, for cake, chicken, pickles. The mother answered his every call like an obedient slave; and when the food called for did not come as soon as was desired, as the cries and calls become unpleasantly urgent, the mother answered, "Yes, yes, darling, you shall have it." After the food was placed in his hand, it was thrown passionately upon the car floor, because it did not come soon enough. *(Health Reformer, December, 1870)*

"Likelihood of a vegetarian reaching the age of 80 compared to a non-vegetarian after adjusting for smoking, 1.8 times greater."

British Medical Journal, 1996; 313:775–79

221

A child of about ten years was afflicted with chills and fever, and was disinclined to eat. The mother urged her: "Eat a little of this sponge cake. Here is some nice chicken. Won't you have a taste of these preserves?" The child finally ate a large meal for a well person. The food urged upon her was not proper for the stomach in health, and should in no case be taken while sick. The mother, in about two hours, was bathing the head of the child, saying she could not understand why she should have such a burning fever. She had added fuel to the fire, and wondered that the fire burned. Had that child been left to let nature take her course, and the stomach take the rest so necessary for it, her sufferings might have been far less. These mothers were not prepared to bring up children. The greatest cause of human suffering is ignorance on the subject of how to treat our own bodies. *(Health Reformer, December, 1870)*

222

I heard parents remark that the appetites of their children were delicate, and unless they had meat and cake, they could not eat. When the noon meal was taken, I observed the quality of food given to these children. It was fine wheaten bread, sliced ham coated with black pepper, spiced pickles, cake, and preserves. The pale, sallow complexion of these children plainly indicated the abuses the stomach was suffering. Two of these children observed another family of children eating cheese with their food, and they lost their appetite for what was before them until their indulgent mother begged a piece of the cheese to give to her children, fearing the dear children would fail to make out their meal. *(Testimonies, Volume 3, 1875)*

223

The cook fills an important place in the household. She is preparing food to be taken into the stomach, to form brain, bone, and muscle. The health of all members of the family depends largely upon her skill and intelligence. Household duties will never receive the attention they demand until those who faithfully perform them are held in proper respect. *(Christian Temperance and Bible Hygiene, 1890)*

"Vegetarian diets decrease the risk of cancer."

World Cancer Research Fund and American Institute for Cancer, "Food, Nutrition and the Prevention of Cancer: A Global Perspective," 1997, 456–57

224

In order to learn how to cook, women should study, and then patiently reduce what they learn to practice. People are suffering because they will not take the trouble to do this. I say to such, It is time for you to rouse your dormant energies, and inform yourselves. Do not think the time wasted which is devoted to obtaining a thorough knowledge and experience in the preparation of healthful, palatable food. No matter how long an experience you have had in cooking, if you still have the responsibilities of a family, it is your duty to learn how to care for them properly. *(Christian Temperance and Bible Hygiene, 1890)*

225

Fathers and mothers, watch unto prayer. Guard strictly against intemperance in every form. Teach your children the principles of true health reform. Teach them what things to avoid in order to preserve health. *(Testimonies, Volume 9, 1909)*

226

*M*any parents educate the tastes of their children, and form their appetites. They indulge them in eating flesh meats, and in drinking tea and coffee. The highly seasoned flesh meats and the tea and coffee, which some mothers encourage their children to use, prepare the way for them to crave stronger stimulants, as tobacco. The use of tobacco encourages the appetite for liquor; and the use of tobacco and liquor invariably lessens nerve power. *(Christian Temperance and Bible Hygiene, 1890)*

227

*I*t is a sin to place poorly prepared food on the table, because the matter of eating concerns the well-being of the entire system. The Lord desires His people to appreciate the necessity of having food prepared in such a way that it will not make sour stomachs, and in consequence, sour tempers. Let us remember that there is practical religion in a loaf of good bread. *(Manuscript Files, 1901)*

"Cow's milk has become a point of controversy among doctors and nutritionists. There was a time when it was considered very desirable, but research has forced us to rethink this recommendation . . . dairy products contribute to a surprising number of health problems."

Benjamin Spock, M.D., *Dr. Spock's Baby and Child Care,* 7th Edition

228

*T*o cook well, to present healthful food upon the table in an inviting manner, requires intelligence and experience. The one who prepares the food that is to be placed in our stomachs, to be converted into blood to nourish the system, occupies a most important and elevated position. *(Testimonies, Volume 3, 1871)*

229

The imprudent eater does not realize that he is disqualifying himself for giving wise counsel. The food he has eaten has benumbed his brain power. *(Manuscript Files, 1901)*

230

Connected with our sanitariums and schools there should be cooking schools, where instruction is given on the proper preparation of food. In all our schools there should be those who are fitted to educate the students, both young men and women, in the art of cooking. *(Manuscript Files, 1901)*

231

Scanty, ill-cooked food depraves the blood by weakening the blood-making organs. It deranges the system, and brings on disease, with its accompaniment of irritable nerves and bad tempers. The victims of poor cookery are numbered by thousands and tens of thousands. Over many graves might be written: 'Died because of poor cooking; Died of an abused stomach.' " *(Ministry of Healing, 1905)*

232

The proper cooking of food is a most important accomplishment. Especially where meat is not made a principal article of food is good cooking an essential requirement. Something must be prepared to take the place of meat, and these substitutes for meat must be well prepared, so that meat will not be desired. *(1896 Letter)*

233

*T*hose who do not know how to cook hygienically should learn to combine wholesome, nourishing articles of food in such a way as to make appetizing dishes. Let those who desire to gain knowledge in this line subscribe for our health journals. They will find information on this point in them. *(1902 Letter)*

"Pancreatic cancer occurs much more frequently in countries where fat consumption and/or animal product consumption is high."

American Journal of Epidemiology, 1990; 132:423–431

234

*M*any who adopt the health reform complain that it does not agree with them; but after sitting at their tables I come to the conclusion that it is not the health reform that is at fault, but the poorly prepared food. I appeal to men and women to whom God has given intelligence: Learn how to cook. I make no mistake when I say "men," for they, as well as women, need to understand the simple, healthful preparation of food. Their business often takes them where they cannot obtain wholesome food. They may be called to remain days and even weeks in families that are entirely ignorant in this respect. Then, if they have the knowledge, they can use it to good purpose. *(Christian Temperance and Bible Hygiene, 1890)*

235

*Y*ou should keep grease out of your food. It defiles any preparation of food you may make. Eat largely of fruits and vegetables. *(Testimonies, Volume 2, 1868)*

236

We need persons who will educate themselves to cook healthfully. Many know how to cook meats and vegetables in different forms, who yet do not understand how to prepare simple and appetizing dishes. *(Youth's Instructor, 1894)*

237

It is important that the food should be prepared with care, that the appetite, when not perverted, can relish it. Because we from principle discard the use of meat, butter, mince pies, spices, lard, and that which irritates the stomach and destroys health, the idea should never be given that it is of but little consequence what we eat. *(Testimonies, Volume 2, 1870)*

> "Those men who are prostate-cancer patients consume a diet higher in fat than those who do not have prostate cancer. When animal product consumption is compared to the rates of death, it is found that the consumption of meat and dairy products correlate very closely with the death rate."
>
> *Cancer, 1989; 64:598–604*

238

For want of knowledge and skill in regard to cooking, many a wife and mother daily sets before her family ill-prepared food, which is steadily and surely impairing the digestive organs, and making a poor quality of blood; the result is, frequent attacks of inflammatory disease, and sometimes death. We can have a variety of good, wholesome food, cooked in a healthful manner, so that it will be palatable to all. It is of vital importance to know how to cook. *(Christian Temperance and Bible Hygiene, 1890)*

239

*I*t is the positive duty of physicians to educate, educate, educate, by pen and voice, all who have the responsibility of preparing food for the table. *(1896 Letter)*

240

*C*ooking is no mean science and it is one of the most essential in practical life. It is a science that all women should learn, and it should be taught in a way to benefit the poorer classes. To make food appetizing and at the same time simple and nourishing, requires skill; but it can be done. Cooks should know how to prepare simple food in a simple and healthful manner, and so that it will be found more palatable, as well as more wholesome, because of its simplicity. Every woman who is at the head of a family and yet does not understand the art of healthful cookery should determine to learn that which is so essential to the well-being of her household. In many places hygienic cooking schools afford opportunity for instruction in this line. She who has not the help of such facilities should put herself under the instruction of some good cook, and persevere in her efforts for improvement until she is mistress of the culinary art. *(Ministry of Healing, 1905)*

241

*I*t is wrong to eat merely to gratify the appetite, but no indifference should be manifested regarding the quality of the food, or the manner of its preparation. If the food eaten is not relished, the body will not be so well nourished. The food should be carefully chosen and prepared with intelligence and skill. *(Ministry of Healing, 1905)*

242

It is sacred duty for those who cook to learn how to prepare healthful food. Many souls are lost as the result of poor cookery. It takes thought and care to make good bread; but there is more religion in a loaf of good bread than may think. There are few really good cooks. Young women think that it is menial to cook and do other kinds of housework; and for this reason, many girls who marry and have the care of families have little idea of the duties devolving upon a wife and mother. *(Ministry of Healing, 1905)*

> "Intervention programs targeting children's dietary fat behaviors should include teaching skills that enable children to ask for low-fat foods . . . These foods should be made available in the home to encourage children to practice low-fat dietary behaviors."
>
> *Journal of the American Dietetic Association,* 2002; 102:1773–1778

243

Animals are becoming more and more diseased, and it will not be long until animal food will be discarded by many besides Seventh-day Adventists. Foods that are healthful and life sustaining are to be prepared, so that men and women will not need to eat meat. *(Testimonies, Volume 7, 1902)*

244

Before children take lessons on the organ or the piano they should be given lessons in cooking. The work of learning to cook need not exclude music, but to learn music is of less importance than to learn how to prepare food that is wholesome and appetizing. *(Testimonies, Volume 1, 1868)*

245

$\mathcal{D}$o not neglect to teach your children how to cook. In doing so, you impart to them principles which they must have in their religious education. In giving your children lessons in physiology, and teaching them how to cook with simplicity and yet with skill, you are laying the foundation for the most useful branches of education. Skill is required to make good light bread. *(Testimonies, Volume 2, 1870)*

246

$\mathcal{T}$here is much to be learned regarding the preparation of healthful foods. Foods that are perfectly healthful and yet inexpensive are to be made. To the poor the gospel of health is to be preached. In the manufacture of these foods, ways will be opened up whereby those who accept the truth and lose their work, will be able to earn a living. *(1901 Letter)*

"Cancer odds ratios for the highest percentiles of red meat intake (7 or more times per week) compared with the lowest (3 or fewer times per week) were 1.6 for stomach, 1.9 for colon, 1.7 for rectal, 1.6 for pancreatic, 1.6 for bladder, 1.2 for breast, 1.5 for endometrial and 1.3 for ovarian cancer."

International Journal of Cancer, May 1, 2000; 86:425–428

247

$\mathcal{S}$killful teachers should show the people how to utilize to the very best advantage the products that they can raise or secure in their section of the country. Thus the poor, as well as those in better circumstances, can learn to live healthfully. *(Testimonies, Volume 7, 1902)*

248

*D*eal in foods that are much less costly, and which, prepared in a nutritious form, will answer every purpose. Endeavor to produce less expensive preparations of the grains and fruits. All these are freely given us of God to supply our necessities. Health is not ensured by the use of expensive preparations. We can have just as good health while using the simple preparations from the fruits, grains, and the vegetables. *(Testimonies, Volume 7, 1902)*

249

*I*t is a religious duty for those who cook to learn how to prepare healthful food in different ways, so that it may be eaten with enjoyment. Mothers should teach their children how to cook. What branch of the education of a young lady can be so important as this? The eating has to do with the life. Scanty, impoverished, ill-cooked food is constantly depraving the blood, by weakening the blood-making organs. It is highly essential that the art of cookery be considered one of the most important branches of education. There are but few good cooks. *(Testimonies, Volume 1, 1868)*

250

*W*hen the message comes to those who have not heard the truth for this time, they see that a great reformation must take place in their diet. They see that they must put away flesh food, because it creates an appetite for liquor and fills the system with disease. By meat eating, the physical, mental, and moral powers are weakened. Man is built up from that which he eats. Animal passions bear sway as the result of meat eating, tobacco using, and liquor drinking. *(Manuscript Files, 1901)*

251

*I*t is our wisdom to prepare simple, inexpensive, healthful foods. Many of our people are poor, and healthful foods are to be provided that can be supplied at prices that the poor can afford to pay. It is the Lord's design that the poorest people in every place shall be supplied with inexpensive, healthful foods. In many places industries for the manufacture of these foods are to be established. That which is a blessing to the work in one place will be a blessing in another place where money is very much harder to obtain. *(Manuscript Files, 1905)*

"A causal relationship between red meat consumption and cancer is supported by several large studies conducted in the U.S. Specifically, women with the highest level of meat consumption had double the rate of breast cancer compared to those who consumed small amounts of meat."

Epidemiology, 5:4 (1994), 391

252

*I*t is the duty of the physician to see that wholesome food is provided, and it should be prepared in a way that will not create disturbances in the human organism. *(Manuscript Files, 1901)*

253

*P*hysicians should watch unto prayer, realizing that they stand in a position of great responsibility. They should prescribe for their patients the food best suited for them. This food should be prepared by one who realizes that he occupies a most important position, inasmuch as good food is required to make good blood. *(1909 Letter)*

254

It is right that no tea, coffee, or flesh meat be served in our sanitariums. To many, this is a great change and a severe deprivation. To enforce other changes, such as a change in the number of meals a day, is likely, in the cases of some, to do more harm than good. *(1904 Letter)*

"Average I.Q. of U.S. children: 97"

Los Angeles Times, Feb 6, 1993

"Average I.Q. of vegetarian children: 116"

Journal of the American Dietetic Association, 1980; 76:142–47

255

An important part of the nurse's duty is the care of the patient's diet. The patient should not be allowed to suffer or became unduly weakened through lack of nourishment, nor should the enfeebled digestive powers be overtaxed. Care should be taken so to prepare and serve the food that it will be palatable, but wise judgment should be used in adapting it to the needs of the patient, both in quantity and quality. *(Ministry of Healing, 1905)*

256

The patients are to be provided with an abundance of wholesome, palatable food, prepared and served in so appetizing a way that they will have no temptation to desire flesh meat. The meals may be made the means of an education in health reform. Care is to be shown in regard to the combinations of food given to the patients. *(1902 Letter)*

257

*A*s the truth is presented in new places, lessons should be given in hygienic cookery. Teach the people how they may live without the use of flesh meats. Teach them the simplicity of living. *(Manuscript Files, 1906)*

258

*T*hese people have lived improperly on rich food. They are suffering as a result of indulgence of appetite. A reform in their habits of eating and drinking is needed. But this reform cannot be made all at once. The change must be made gradually. The health foods set before them must be appetizing. All their lives, perhaps, they have had three meals a day, and have eaten rich food. It is an important matter to reach these people with the truths of health reform. But in order to lead them to adopt a sensible diet, you must set before them an abundant supply of wholesome, appetizing food. Changes must not be made so abruptly that they will be turned from health reform, instead of being led to it. The food served to them must be nicely prepared, and it must be richer than either you or I would eat. *(1904 Letter)*

"We assessed the effect of a diet high in leafy and green vegetables, fruit, and nuts on serum lipid risk factors for cardiovascular disease. After 2 weeks on the vegetable diet, lipid risk factors for cardiovascular disease were significantly reduced. On the vegetable compared with the control diet, the reduction in total serum cholesterol was 34% to 49% greater than would be predicted by differences in dietary fat and cholesterol. A diet consisting largely of low-calorie vegetables and fruit and nuts markedly reduced lipid risk factors for cardiovascular disease."

Metabolism, 1997 May; 46(5):530–7

259

Let fruit be placed on the table in abundance. *(1902 Letter)*

260

Physicians who use flesh meat and prescribe it for their
patients, should not be employed in our institutions, because
they fail decidedly in educating the patients to discard that which
makes them sick. The physician who uses and prescribes meat
does not reason from cause to effect, and instead of acting as
a restorer, he leads the patient by his own example to indulge
perverted appetite. The physicians employed in our institutions
should be reformers in this respect and in every other. Many of
the patients are suffering because of errors in diet. They need to
be shown the better way. But how can a meat-eating physician
do this? By his wrong habits he trammels his work and cripples
his usefulness. *(1896 Letter)*

261

I remember once, when at the sanitarium, I was urged to
sit at the table with the patients, and eat with them, that we
might become acquainted. I saw then that a decided mistake was
being made in the preparation of the food. It was put together
in such a way that it was tasteless, and there was not more than
two thirds enough. I found it impossible to make a meal that
would satisfy my appetite. *(1904 Letter)*

"Populations of vegetarians living in affluent countries appear to
enjoy unusually good health, characterized by low rates of cancer,
cardiovascular disease, and total mortality."

American Journal of Clinical Nutrition, 1999 Sep; 70 (3 Suppl):434S–438S

262

*I*n all our sanitariums a liberal bill of fare should be arranged for the patients' dining room. I have not seen anything very extravagant in any of our medical institutions; but I have seen some tables that were decidedly lacking in a supply of good, inviting, palatable food. Often patients at such institutions, after remaining for a while, have decided that they were paying a large sum for room, board, and treatment, without receiving much in return, and have therefore left. Of course, complaints greatly to the discredit of the institution were soon in circulation. *(1904 Letter)*

263

*T*he men and women of the world who come to our sanitariums often have perverted appetites. Radical changes cannot be made suddenly for all these. Some cannot at once be placed on as plain a health reform diet as would be acceptable in a private family. In a medical institution there are varied appetites to satisfy. Some require well-prepared vegetables to meet their peculiar needs. *(1904 Letter)*

264

*T*hose who come to our sanitariums for treatment should be provided with a liberal supply of well-cooked food. The food placed before them must necessarily be more varied in kind than would be necessary in a home family. Let the diet be such that a good impression will be made on the guests. This is a matter of great importance. The patronage of a sanitarium will be larger if a liberal supply of appetizing food is provided. *(Manuscript Files, 1901)*

265

We must remember that the habits and practices of a lifetime cannot be changed in a moment. With an intelligent cook, and an abundant supply of wholesome food, reforms can be brought about that will work well. But it may take time to bring them about. *(1904 Letter)*

266

There needs to be presented to all students and physicians, and by them to others, that the whole animal creation is more or less diseased. Diseased meat is not rare, but common. Every phase of disease is brought into the human system through subsisting upon the flesh of dead animals. *(1903 Letter)*

267

This meat-eating question needs to be guarded. When one changes from the stimulating diet of meat eating to the fruit-and-vegetable diet, there will always be at first a sense of weakness and of lack of vitality, and many urge this as an argument for the necessity of a meat diet. But this result is the very argument that should be used in discarding a meat diet. *(1896 Letter)*

268

When a physician sees a patient suffering from disease caused by improper eating and drinking or other wrong habits, yet neglects to tell him of this, he is doing his fellow being an injury. Those who understand the principles of life should be in earnest in striving to counteract the causes of disease. *(Ministry of Healing, 1905)*

269

Let those who are sick do all in their power, by correct practice in eating, drinking, and dressing, and by taking judicious exercise, to secure recovery of health. *(1890 Letter)*

"It is found that, given a constant calcium intake, a twofold increase in dietary protein high in sulfur amino acids (such as that found in animal products) produces a 50% increase in urinary calcium loss. In contrast, a diet rich in soy protein does not promote calcium loss."

American Journal of Clinical Nutrition, 48, 1988

270

Indulging in eating too frequently and in too large quantities, overtaxes the digestive organs and produces a feverish state of the system. The blood becomes impure, and then diseases of various kinds occur. A physician is sent for, who prescribes some drug which gives present relief, but which does not cure the disease. It may change the form of disease, but the real evil is increased tenfold. Nature was doing her best to rid the system of an accumulation of impurities, and could she have been left to herself, aided by the common blessings of Heaven, such as pure air and pure water, a speedy and safe cure would have been effected. The sufferers in such cases can do for themselves that which others cannot do as well for them. They should commence to relieve nature of the load they have forced upon her. They should remove the cause. Fast a short time, and give the stomach chance for rest. Reduce the feverish state of the system by a careful and understanding application of water. These efforts will help nature in her struggles to free the system of impurities. *(Spiritual Gifts, Book 4, 1864)*

"The matched subjects who ate meat (including poultry and fish) were more than twice as likely to become demented as their vegetarian counterparts."

Neuroepidemiology, 1993; 12(1):28–36

271

Every person should have a knowledge of nature's remedial agencies and how to apply them. It is essential both to understand the principles involved in the treatment of the sick and to have a practical training that will enable one rightly to use this knowledge. The use of natural remedies requires an amount of care and effort that many are not willing to give. Nature's process of healing and up-building is gradual, and to the impatient it seems slow. The surrender of hurtful indulgences requires sacrifice. But in the end it will be found that nature, untrammeled, does her work wisely and well. Those who persevere in obedience to her laws will reap the reward in health of body and health of mind. *(Ministry of Healing, 1905)*

272

Physicians often advise invalids to visit foreign countries, to go to some mineral spring, or to traverse the ocean, in order to regain health; when, in nine cases out of ten, if they would eat temperately, and engage in healthful exercise with a cheerful spirit, they would regain health and save time and money. Exercise, and a free, abundant use of the air and sunlight— blessings which heaven has bestowed upon all—would in many cases give life and strength to the emaciated invalid. *(Christian Temperance and Bible Hygiene, 1890)*

273

*P*ure air and water, cleanliness, a proper diet, purity of life, and a firm trust in God, are remedies for the want of which thousands are dying; yet these remedies are going out of date because their skilful use requires work that the people do not appreciate. Fresh air, exercise, pure water, and clean, sweet premises, are within the reach of all, with but little expense; but drugs are expensive, both in the outlay of means, and the effect produced upon the system. *(Testimonies, Volume 5, 1885)*

274

*I*n regard to that which we can do for ourselves, there is a point that requires careful, thoughtful consideration. I must become acquainted with myself, I must be a learner always as to how to take care of this building, the body God has given me, that I may preserve it in the very best condition of health. I must eat those things which will be for my very best good physically, and I must take special care to have my clothing such as will conduce to a healthful circulation of the blood. I must not deprive myself of exercise and air. I must have wisdom to be a faithful guardian of my body. *(1904 Letter)*

275

*I*f you regard your life, you should eat plain food, prepared in the simplest manner, and take more physical exercise. Each member of the family needs the benefits of health reform. But drugging should be forever abandoned; for while it does not cure any malady, it enfeebles the system, making it more susceptible to disease. *(Testimonies, Volume 5, 1885)*

276

It was presented to me that we should not rest satisfied because we have a vegetarian restaurant in Brooklyn, but that others should be established in other sections of the city. Men and women who eat at the restaurants established in different places will become conscious of an improvement in health. Their confidence once gained, they will be more ready to accept God's special message of truth. Wherever medical missionary work is carried on in our large cities, cooking schools should be held; and wherever a strong educational missionary work is in progress, a hygienic restaurant of some sort should be established, which shall give a practical illustration of the proper selection and the healthful preparation of foods. *(Testimonies, Volume 7, 1902)*

277

The more we depend upon the fresh fruit just as it is plucked from the tree, the greater will be the blessing. *(Testimonies, Volume 7, 1902)*

"High-vegetable fiber intakes reduce risk factors for cardiovascular disease and possibly colon cancer."

Metabolism, 2001 Apr; 50(4):494–503

278

It would be well for us to do less cooking and to eat more fruit in its natural state. Let us teach the people to eat freely of the fresh grapes, apples, peaches, pears, berries, and all other kinds of fruit that can be obtained. Let these be prepared for winter use by canning, using glass, as far as possible, instead of tin. *(Testimonies, Volume 2, 1870)*

279

The question of health reform is not agitated as it must and will be. A simple diet, and the entire absence of drugs, leaving nature free to recuperate the wasted energies of the body, would make our sanitariums far more effectual in restoring the sick to health. *(1896 Letter)*

280

Many are living in violation of the laws of health, and are ignorant of the relation their habits of eating, drinking, and working sustain to their health. They will not arouse to their true condition until nature protests against the abuses she is suffering, by aches and pains in the system. If, even then, the sufferers would only commence the work right, and would resort to the simple means they have neglected,—the use of water and proper diet,—nature would have just the help she requires, and which she ought to have had long before. If this course is pursued, the patient will generally recover without being debilitated. *(Spiritual Gifts, Book 4, 1864)*

281

For a dyspeptic stomach, you may place upon your tables fruits of different kinds, but not too many at one meal. *(Testimonies, Volume 7, 1902)*

"Type 2 diabetes mellitus is much less likely to be a cause of death in vegetarians than non-vegetarians, perhaps because of their higher intake of complex carbohydrates and lower body mass."

American Journal of Clinical Nutrition, 1988; 48 (supplement):712–738

282

*F*ruit we would especially recommend as a health-giving agency. But even fruit should not be eaten after a full meal of other foods. *(Manuscript Files, 1908)*

283

*W*herever fruit can be grown in abundance, a liberal supply should be prepared for winter, by canning or drying. Small fruits, such as currants, gooseberries, strawberries, raspberries, and blackberries, can be grown to advantage in many places where they are but little used, and their cultivation is neglected. Use little sugar, and cook the fruit only long enough to ensure its preservation. Thus prepared, it is an excellent substitute for fresh fruit. *(Ministry of Healing, 1905)*

284

*I*n our medical institutions clear instruction should be given in regard to temperance. The patients should be shown the evil of intoxicating liquor, and the blessing of total abstinence. They should be asked to discard the things that have ruined their health, and the place of these things should be supplied with an abundance of fruit. Oranges, lemons, prunes, peaches, and many other varieties can be obtained; for the Lord's world is productive, if painstaking effort is put forth. *(1904 Letter)*

"Plasma homocysteine levels have been directly associated with cardiac disease risk. We report our observations of homocysteine levels in 40 self selected subjects who participated in a vegan diet-based lifestyle program. Subjects' mean homocysteine levels fell 13%."

Preventive Medicine, 2000 Mar; 30(3):225–233

285

Our diet should be suited to the season, to the climate in which we live, and to the occupation we follow. Some foods that are adapted for use at one season or in one climate are not suited to another. *(Ministry of Healing, 1905)*

286

Do not eat largely of salt, avoid the use of pickles and spiced foods, eat an abundance of fruit, and the irritation that calls for so much drink at mealtime will largely disappear. *(Ministry of Healing, 1905)*

287

If you can get apples, you are in a good condition as far as fruit is concerned, if you have nothing else. Apples are superior to any fruit for a standby that grows. *(1870 Letter)*

288

Applesauce, put up in glass, is wholesome and palatable. Pears and cherries, if they can be obtained, make very nice sauce for winter use. *(1905 Letter)*

289

A diet lacking in the proper elements of nutrition brings reproach upon the cause of health reform. We are mortal, and must supply ourselves with food that will give proper sustenance to the body. *(1902 Letter)*

290

ℱamilies and institutions should learn to do more in the cultivation and improvement of land. If people only knew the value of the products of the ground, which the earth brings forth in their season, more diligent efforts would be made to cultivate the soil. All should be acquainted with the special value of fruits and vegetables fresh from the orchard and garden. *(Manuscript Files, 1911)*

291

ℐf we plan wisely, that which is most conducive to health can be secured in almost every land. The various preparations of rice, wheat, corn, and oats are sent abroad everywhere, also beans, peas, and lentils. These, with native or imported fruits, and the variety of vegetables that grow in each locality, give an opportunity to select a dietary that is complete without the use of flesh meats. *(Ministry of Healing, 1905)*

292

𝒲hen flesh food is discarded, its place should be supplied with a variety of grains, nuts, vegetables, and fruits, that will be both nourishing and appetizing. The place of meat should be supplied with wholesome foods that are inexpensive. *(Ministry of Healing, 1905)*

"Fecal sulfide concentrations were significantly related to meat intake. Dietary protein from meat is an important substrate for sulfide generation by bacteria in the human large intestine."

American Journal of Clinical Nutrition, 2000 Dec; 72(6):1488–94

293

*B*read should be thoroughly baked, inside and out. The health of the stomach demands that it be light and dry. Bread is the real staff of life, and therefore every cook should excel in making it. *(Manuscript Files, 1899)*

294

*H*ot soda biscuits are often spread with butter, and eaten as a choice diet; but the enfeebled digestive organs cannot but feel the abuse placed upon them. *(1896 Letter)*

295

*A*ll wheat flour is not best for a continuous diet. A mixture of wheat, oatmeal, and rye would be more nutritious than the wheat with the nutrifying properties separated from it. *(1898 Letter)*

296

*S*weet breads and cookies we seldom have on our table. The less of sweet foods that are eaten, the better; these cause disturbances in the stomach, and produce impatience and irritability in those who accustom themselves to their use. *(1907 Letter)*

297

*T*he Lord intends to bring His people back to live upon simple fruits, vegetables, and grains. *(1896 Letter)*

298

*I*t is an error generally committed to make no difference in the life of a woman previous to the birth of her children. Great changes are going on in her system. It requires a greater amount of blood, and therefore, and increase of food of the most nourishing quality. *(Testimonies, Volume 2, 1870)*

"We conclude that grilled red meat intake is a risk factor for pancreatic cancer and that method of meat preparation in addition to total intake is important in assessing the effects of meat consumption in epidemiologic studies."

Mutation Research, September 2002, Volume 506–507

299

*F*or use in bread making, the superfine white flour is not the best. Its use is neither healthful nor economical. Fine-flour bread is lacking in nutritive elements to be found in bread made from the whole wheat. It is a frequent cause of constipation and other unhealthful conditions. *(Ministry of Healing, 1905)*

300

*I*t is well to leave sugar out of the crackers that are made. Some enjoy best the sweetest crackers, but these are an injury to the digestive organs. *(1901 Letter)*

301

*T*he simple grains, fruits of the trees, vegetables, have all the nutritive properties necessary to make good blood. This a flesh diet cannot do. *(1896 Letter)*

302

𝐴 variety of simple dishes, perfectly healthful and nourishing, may be provided, aside from meat. Hearty men must have plenty of vegetables, fruits, and grains. *(1884 Letter)*

303

𝐴nother very simple yet wholesome dish, is beans boiled or baked. *(Testimonies, Volume 2, 1871)*

304

𝑊hen I went to see the sick man, I tired to tell them as well as I could how to manage, and soon he began slowly to improve. But he imprudently exercised his strength when not able, ate a small amount not of the right quality, and was taken down again. This time there was no help for him. His system appeared to be a living mass of corruption. He died a victim to poor cooking. He tried to make sugar supply the place of good cooking, and it only made matters worse. *(Testimonies, Volume 2, 1870)*

"Vegans tend to have low serum lipids, lean physiques, shorter stature, later puberty, and decreased risk for certain prominent 'Western' cancers; a vegan diet has documented clinical efficacy in rheumatoid arthritis. Low-fat vegan diets may be especially protective in regard to cancers linked to insulin resistance—namely, breast and colon cancer—as well as prostate cancer; conversely, the high IGF-I activity associated with heavy ingestion of animal products may be largely responsible for the epidemic of 'Western' cancers in wealthy societies. Increased phytochemical intake is also likely to contribute to the reduction of cancer risk in vegans."

Medical Hypotheses, 1999 Dec; 53(6):459–85

305

I would advise all to take something warm into the stomach, every morning at least. You can do this without much labor. *(Testimonies, Volume 2, 1870)*

306

*P*rovision should be made for obtaining a supply of dried sweet corn. Pumpkins can be dried, and used to advantage during the winter in making pies. *(1905 Letter)*

307

*T*he tomatoes you sent were very nice and very palatable. I find that tomatoes are the best article of diet for me to use. *(1900 Letter)*

308

*O*f corn and peas we have raised enough for ourselves and our neighbors. The sweet corn we dry for winter use; then when we need it we grind it in a mill and cook it. It makes most palatable soups and other dishes. In their season we have grapes in abundance, also prunes and apples, and some cherries, peaches, pears, and olives, which we prepare ourselves. *(1907 Letter)*

309

*M*any do not see the importance of having land to cultivate, and of raising fruit and vegetables, that their tables may be supplied with these things. *(1904 Letter)*

310

Anything that hinders the active motion of the living machinery, affects the brain very directly. And from the light given me, sugar, when largely used, is more injurious than meat. These changes should be made cautiously, and the subject should be treated in a manner not calculated to disgust and prejudice those whom we would teach and help. *(Testimonies, Volume 2, 1870)*

"Nine studies of childhood brain tumors and maternal diet during pregnancy have focused on foods. An association between frequent consumption of cured meat by pregnant women and increased risk is a consistent finding in most of the studies."

International Journal of Cancer, Suppl. 1998; 11:23–5

311

Sugar is not good for the stomach. It causes fermentation, and this clouds the brain and brings peevishness into the disposition. *(Manuscript Files, 1901)*

312

At too many tables, when the stomach has received all that it requires to properly carry on its work of nourishing the system, another course, consisting of pies, puddings, and highly flavored sauces, is placed upon the table. Many, though they have already eaten enough, will overstep the bounds, and eat the tempting dessert, which, however, proves anything but good for them. If the extras which are provided for dessert were dispensed with altogether, it would be a blessing. *(Christian Temperance and Bible Hygiene, 1890)*

313

*N*ow in regard to milk and sugar: Large quantities of milk and sugar eaten together are injurious. They impart impurities to the system. Animals from which milk is obtained are not always healthy. They may be diseased. A cow may be apparently well in the morning and die before night. Then she was diseased in the morning, and her milk was diseased, but you did not know it. The animal creation is diseased. Flesh meats are diseased. Could we know that animals were in perfect health, I would recommend that people eat flesh meats sooner than large quantities of milk and sugar. It would not do the injury that milk and sugar do. *(Testimonies, Volume 2, 1870)*

314

*S*ugar clogs the system. It hinders the working of the living machine. *(Testimonies, Volume 2, 1870)*

315

*E*verything is plain yet wholesome because it is not merely thrown together in a haphazard manner. We have no sugar on our table. Our sauce which is our dependence is apples, baked or stewed, sweetened as is required before being put upon the table. *(1870 Letter)*

"The administration of subtherapeutic doses of antibiotics to livestock introduces selective pressures that may lead to the emergence and dissemination of resistant bacteria. The present findings clearly demonstrate that antibiotic-resistant bacteria in beef and milk pose a serious problem."

Journal of Food Protein, 1999 June, 62:6

316

I frequently sit down to the tables of the brethren and sisters, and see that they use a great amounts of milk and sugar. These clog the system, irritate the digestive organs, and affect the brain. *(Testimonies, Volume 2, 1870)*

317

*T*he human family have indulged an increasing desire for rich food, until it has become a fashion to crowd all the delicacies possible into the stomach. Especially at parties of pleasure is the appetite indulged with but little restraint. Rich dinners and late suppers are partaken of, consisting of highly seasoned meats with rich gravies, rich cakes, pies, ice cream, etc. *(Spiritual Gifts, Book 4, 1864)*

318

*T*he light given me is that a most decided message must be borne in regard to health reform. Those who use flesh meat strengthen the lower propensities and prepare the way for disease to fasten upon them. *(1903 Letter)*

319

*B*ecause it is the fashion, in harmony with morbid appetite, rich cake, pies, and puddings, and every hurtful thing, are crowded into the stomach. The table must be loaded down with a variety, or the depraved appetite cannot be satisfied. In the morning, these slaves to appetite often have impure breath, and a furred tongue. They do not enjoy health, and wonder why they suffer with pains, headaches, and various ills. *(1896 Letter)*

"The lifetime risk of ischemic heart disease (IHD) was reduced by approximately 31% in those who consumed nuts frequently and by 37% in male vegetarians compared with non-vegetarians. Cancers of the colon and prostate were significantly more likely in non-vegetarians, and frequent beef consumers also had higher risk of bladder cancer. Intake of legumes was negatively associated with risk of colon cancer in non-vegetarians and risk of pancreatic cancer. Higher consumption of all fruit or dried fruit was associated with lower risks of lung, prostate, and pancreatic cancers."

American Journal of Clinical Nutrition, 1999 Sep; 70 (3 Suppl):532S–538S

320

Especially harmful are the custards and puddings in which milk, eggs, and sugar are the chief ingredients. The free use of milk and sugar taken together should be avoided. *(Fundamentals of Christian Education, October, 1893)*

321

Because it is fashion, many who are poor and dependent upon their daily labor, will be to the expense of preparing different kinds of rich cakes, preserves, pies, and a variety of fashionable food for visitors, which only injure those who partake of them; when, at the same time, they need the amount thus expended, to purchase clothing for themselves and children. *(How to Live, Book 1, 1865)*

322

The victim of appetite is so wedded to his own way that he cannot see the injury he is doing to himself. *(1895 Letter)*

323

*M*any understand how to make different kinds of cakes, but cake is not the best food to be placed upon the table. Sweet cakes, sweet puddings, and custards will disorder the digestive organs; and why should we tempt those who surround the table by placing such articles before them? *(How to Live, Book 1, 1865)*

324

*T*he desserts which take so much time to prepare, are detrimental to health. *(Christian Temperance and Bible Hygiene, 1890. Youth's Instructor, May 31, 1894)*

325

*F*lesh meats and rich cakes and pies prepared with spices of any kind, are not the most healthful and nourishing diet. *(Testimonies, Volume 2, 1870)*

"Oxidative damage is thought to represent one of the mechanisms leading to chronic diseases such atherosclerosis and cancer. Many studies suggest that a link exists between fruit and vegetables in the diet or the amounts of plasma antioxidant vitamins and risk of death from cancer or coronary heart diseases."
European Journal of Cancer Prevention, 1997 Mar; 6 Suppl 1:S15

326

*T*he dessert should be placed on the table and served with the rest of the food; for often, after the stomach has been given all it should have, the dessert is brought on, and is just that much too much. *(1898 Letter)*

327

ƒar too much sugar is ordinarily used in food. Cakes, sweet puddings, pastries, jellies, jams, are active causes of indigestion. *(Ministry of Healing, 1905)*

328

The inflamed condition of the drunkard's stomach is often pictured as illustrating the effect of alcoholic liquors. A similarly inflamed condition is produced by the use of irritating condiments. Soon ordinary food does not satisfy the appetite. The system feels a want, a craving, for something more stimulating. *(Ministry of Healing, 1905)*

329

Under the head of stimulants and narcotics is classed a great variety of articles that, altogether, used as food or drink irritate the stomach, poison the blood, and excite the nerves. Their use is a positive evil. Men seek the excitement of stimulants, because, for the time, the results are agreeable. But there is always a reaction. The use of unnatural stimulants always tends to excess, and it is an active agent in promoting physical degeneration and decay. *(Ministry of Healing, 1905)*

"Studies have suggested that bovine serum albumin is the milk protein responsible for the onset of diabetes . . . Patients with insulin-dependent diabetes mellitus produce antibodies to cow milk proteins that participate in the development of islet dysfunction . . . Taken as a whole, our findings suggest that an active response in patients with IDDM (to the bovine protein) is a feature of the autoimmune response."

New England Journal of Medicine, July 30, 1992

330

*A*s intelligent human beings, let us individually study the principles, and use our experience and judgment in deciding what foods are best for us. *(Testimonies, Volume 7, 1902)*

331

*T*he weakness you experience without the use of meat is one of the strongest arguments I could present to you as a reason why you should discontinue its use. Those who eat meat feel stimulated after eating this food, and they suppose they are made stronger. After one discontinues the use of meat, he may for a time feel a weakness, but when his system is cleansed from the effect of this diet, he no longer feels the weakness, and will cease to wish for that which he has pleaded for as essential to his strength. *(1896 Letter)*

332

*L*et health reformers remember that they may do harm by publishing recipes which do not recommend health reform. Great care is to be shown in furnishing recipes for custards and pastry. If for dessert sweet cake is eaten with milk or cream, fermentation will be created in the stomach, and then the weak points of the human organism will tell the story. The brain will be affected by the disturbance in the stomach. This may be easily cured if people will study from cause to effect, cutting out of their diet that which injures the digestive organs and causes pain in the head. By unwise eating, men and women are unfitted for the work they might do without injury to themselves if they would eat simply. *(1900 Letter)*

333

I wish we were all health reformers. I am opposed to the use of pastries. These mixtures are unhealthful; no one can have good digestive powers and a clear brain who will eat largely of sweet cookies and cream cake and all kinds of pies, and partake of a great variety of food at one meal. When we do this, and then take cold, the whole system is so clogged and enfeebled that it has no power of resistance, no strength to combat disease. I would prefer a meat diet to the sweet cakes and pastries so generally used. *(1891 Letter)*

334

*T*he desserts that are taken in the form of custards are liable to do more harm than good. Fruit, if it can be obtained, is the best article of food. *(1898 Letter)*

335

*I*t is better to let sweet things alone. Let alone those sweet dessert dishes that are placed on the table. You do not need them. *(Review and Herald, January 7, 1902)*

"Many foods, particularly plant foods, contain substances that may have health promoting properties."

British Medical Bulletin, 2000; 56(1):18–33

336

*C*ondiments, so frequently used by those of the world, are ruinous to the digestion. *(1900 Letter)*

337

Condiments and spices used in the preparation of food for the table aid in digestion in the same way that tea, coffee, and liquor are supposed to help the laboring man perform his tasks. After the immediate effects are gone, they drop as correspondingly below par as they were elevated above par by these stimulating substances. The system is weakened. The blood is contaminated, and inflammation is the sure result. *(Excerpts From Unpublished Testimonies in Regard to Flesh Food, 1896)*

338

Our tables should bear only the most wholesome food, free from every irritating substance. The appetite for liquor is encouraged by the preparation of food with condiments and spices. These cause a feverish state of the system, and drink is demanded to allay the irritation. Such is the food that is commonly served upon fashionable tables, and given to the children. Its effect is to cause nervousness and to create thirst which water does not quench. Food should be prepared in as simple a manner as possible, free from condiments and spices, and even from an undue amount of salt. *(Review and Herald, November 6, 1883)*

339

The stomach, after rest and sleep, was better able to take care of a substantial meal than when wearied with work. Then the noon meal was generally soup, sometimes meat. The stomach is small, but the appetite, unsatisfied, partakes largely of this liquid food; so it is burdened. *(1887 Letter)*

340

Spices at first irritate the tender coating of the stomach, but finally destroy the natural sensitiveness of this delicate membrane. The blood becomes fevered, the animal propensities are aroused, while the moral and intellectual powers are weakened, and become servants to the baser passions. The mother should study to set a simple yet nutritious diet before her family. *(Christian Temperance and Bible Hygiene, 1890)*

"Analyses of study data showed that vegans had lower total and LDL cholesterol concentrations than did meat eaters."

American Journal of Clinical Nutrition, 1999 Sep; 70 (3 Suppl):525S–531S

341

Some have so indulged their taste, that unless they have the very article of food it calls for, they find no pleasure in eating. If condiments and spiced foods are placed before them, they make the stomach work by applying this fiery whip; for it has been so treated that it will not acknowledge un-stimulating food. *(1896 Letter)*

342

Luxurious dishes are placed before the children,— spiced foods, rich gravies, cakes, and pastries. This highly seasoned food irritates the stomach, and causes a craving for still stronger stimulants. Not only is the appetite tempted with unsuitable food, of which the children are allowed to eat freely at their meals, but they are permitted to eat between meals; and by the time they are twelve or fourteen years of age, they are often confirmed dyspeptics. *(Christian Temperance and Bible Hygiene, 1890)*

343

$\mathcal{P}$ersons who have indulged their appetite to eat freely of meat, highly seasoned gravies, and various kinds of rich cakes and preserves, cannot immediately relish a plain, wholesome, nutritious diet. Their taste is so perverted they have not appetite for a wholesome diet of fruits, plain bread, and vegetables. They need not expect to relish at first food so different from that in which they have been indulging themselves to eat. *(Spiritual Gifts, Book 4, 1864)*

344

$\mathcal{W}$ith all the precious light that has continually been given to us in the health publications, we cannot afford to live careless, heedless lives, eating and drinking as we please, and indulging in the use of stimulants, narcotics, and condiments. *(Manuscript Files, 1909)*

345

$\mathcal{T}$he use of soda or baking powder in bread making is harmful and unnecessary. Soda causes inflammation of the stomach, and often poisons the entire system. Many housewives think that they cannot make good bread without soda, but this is an error. If they would take the trouble to learn better methods, their bread would be more wholesome, and, to a natural taste, it would be more palatable. *(Ministry of Healing, 1905)*

"Vegetarians have a lower risk of dying from ischemic heart disease than non-vegetarians."

Public Health Nutrition, 1998 Mar; 1(1):33–41

346

People who have a sour stomach are very often of a sour disposition. Everything seems to be contrary to them, and they are inclined to be peevish and irritable. If we would have peace among ourselves, we should give more thought than we do to having a peaceful stomach. *(Manuscript Files, 1908)*

347

Food should be prepared in such a way that it will be appetizing as well as nourishing. It should not be robbed of that which the system needs. I use some salt, and always have, because salt, instead of being deleterious, is actually essential for the blood. *(Testimonies, Volume 9, 1909)*

348

The mince pies and the pickles, which should never find a place in any human stomach, will give a miserable quality of blood. *(Testimonies, Volume 2, 1870)*

349

I was seated once at the table with several children under twelve years of age. Meat was plentifully served, and then a delicate, nervous girl called for pickles. A bottle of chow-chow, fiery with mustard and pungent with spices, was handed her, from which she helped herself freely. The child was proverbial for her nervousness and irritability of temper, and these fiery condiments were well calculated to produce such a condition. *(Christian Temperance and Bible Hygiene, 1890)*

"Food, particularly dairy products, meat, and fish, has been identified as the primary immediate source of intake of polychlorinated dibenzo-p-dioxins (PCDDs), polychlorinated dibenzofurans (PCDFs), and polychlorinated biphenyls (PCBs) for the general population. In addition to the meat, dairy, and fish samples, a vegan (all vegetable, fruit and grain, no animal product) diet, was simulated; this showed the lowest level of dioxins."

Chemosphere, 1997 Mar-Apr; 34(5–7):1437–47

350

*I*n this fast age, the less exciting the food, the better. Condiments are injurious in their nature. Mustard, pepper, spices, pickles, and other things of a like character irritate the stomach and make the blood feverish and impure. *(Ministry of Healing, 1905)*

351

*T*he salads are prepared with oil and vinegar, fermentation takes place in the stomach, and the food does not digest, but decays or putrefies; as a consequence, the blood is not nourished, but becomes filled with impurities, and liver and kidney difficulties appear. *(Testimonies, Volume 2, 1870)*

352

*W*hen properly prepared, olives, like nuts, supply the place of butter and flesh meats. The oil, as eaten in the olive, is far preferable to animal oil or fat. It serves as a laxative. Its use will be found beneficial to consumptives, and it is healing to an inflamed, irritated stomach. *(Ministry of Healing, 1905)*

353

The blood-making organs cannot convert spices, mince pies, pickles, and diseased flesh meats into good blood. *(Ministry of Healing, 1905)*

354

Let the diet reform be progressive. Let the people be taught how to prepare food without the use of milk or butter. Tell them that the time will soon come when there will be no safety in using eggs, milk, cream, or butter, because disease in animals is increasing in proportion to the increase of wickedness among men. The time is near when, because of the iniquity of the fallen race, the whole animal creation will groan under the diseases that curse our earth. *(Testimonies, Volume 7, 1902)*

355

Dumb animals would never eat such a mixture as is often placed in the human stomach. The richness of food and complicated mixtures of food are health destroying. *(1896 Letter)*

356

Olives may be so prepared as to be eaten with good results at every meal. The advantages sought by the use of butter may be obtained by the eating of properly prepared olives. The oil in the olives relieves constipation, and for consumptives, and for those who have inflamed, irritated stomachs, it is better than any drug. As a food it is better than any oil coming secondhand from animals. *(Testimonies, Volume 7, 1902)*

"The majority of toxic dioxin is and (or) has been derived from industrial chlorination processes, incineration of municipal waste, and production of certain herbicides. The lipophilic nature of dioxins results in higher concentrations in the fat of animal and fish products, and their excretion via milk secretion in dairy cattle may result in relatively high concentrations of dioxin contamination in high-fat dairy products."

Journal of Animal Science, 1998 Jan, 76:1

357

The health food business is in need of means and of the active cooperation of our people, that it may accomplish the work it ought to do. Its purpose is to supply the people with food which will take the place of flesh meat, and also milk and butter, which, on account of the diseases of cattle, are becoming more and more objectionable. *(Australasian Union Conference Record, January 1, 1900)*

358

A plain diet, free from spices and flesh meats and grease of all kinds, would prove a blessing to you, and would save your wife a great amount of suffering, grief, and despondency. *(Testimonies, Volume 2, 1868)*

359

Let all who sit down at your table see upon it well-cooked, hygienic, palatable food. Be very careful in regard to your eating and drinking, so that you will not continue to have a diseased body. Eat regularly, and eat only food that is free from grease. *(1904 Letter)*

360

Children are allowed to eat flesh meats, spices, butter, cheese, pork, rich pastry, and condiments generally. They are also allowed to eat irregularly and between meals of unhealthful food. These things do their work of deranging the stomach, exciting the nerves to unnatural action, and enfeebling the intellect. Parents do not realize that they are sowing the seed which will bring forth disease and death. *(Testimonies, Volume 3, 1873)*

361

Many do not feel that this is a matter of duty, hence they do not try to prepare food properly. This can be done in a simple, healthful, and easy manner, without the use of lard, butter, or flesh meats. Skill must be united with simplicity. To do this, women must read, and then patiently reduce what they read to practice. *(Testimonies, Volume 1, 1868)*

"Very high protein intake is known to encourage urinary calcium losses and has been linked to increased fracture risk."

Calcification Tissue International, 1992; 50:14–18

362

The Stomach, when we lie down to rest, should have its work all done, that it may enjoy rest. The work of digestion should not be carried on through any period of the sleeping hours. After the stomach, which has been overtaxed, has performed its task, it becomes exhausted, which causes faintness. Here many are deceived, and think that it is the want of food which produces such feelings, and without giving the stomach time to rest, they take more food. *(How to Live, Book 1, 1865)*

363

$\mathcal{T}$he light given me is that it will not be very long before we shall have to give up any animal food. Even milk will have to be discarded. Disease is accumulating rapidly. The curse of God is upon the earth, because man has cursed it. *(Australasian Union Conference Record, July 28, 1899)*

364

$\mathcal{G}$od wants the perceptive faculties of His people to be clear and capable of hard work. But if you are living on a flesh diet, you need not expect that your mind will be fruitful. The thoughts must be cleansed; then the blessing of God will rest upon His people. *(General Conference Bulletin, April 12, 1901)*

365

$\mathcal{N}$ature is burdened, and endeavors to resist your efforts to cripple her. Chills and fevers are the result of those attempts to rid herself of the burden you lay upon her. You have to suffer the penalty of nature's violated laws. God has established laws in your system which you cannot violate without suffering the punishment. *(Testimonies, Volume 6, 1900)*

366

$\mathcal{Y}$our animal passions should be starved, not pampered and fed. The congestion of blood in the brain is strengthening the animal instincts and weakening spiritual powers. What you need is less temporal food and much more spiritual food, more of the bread of life. The simpler your diet, the better it will be for you. *(1908 Letter)*

"Diets that are rich in plant-derived foods can promote longevity."
Journal of Nutrition, 2003 Jan; 133(1):199–204

367

I eat but two meals a day, and still follow the light given me thirty-five years ago. I use no meat. As for myself, I have settled the butter question. I do not use it. *(1903 Letter)*

368

*N*ature's abundant supply of fruits, nuts, and grains is ample, and year by year the products of all lands are more generally distributed to all, by the increased facilities for transportation. *(Ministry of Healing, 1905)*

369

*M*uch time should be spent in learning how to prepare nut foods. But care should be taken not to reduce the bill of fare to a few articles, using little else than the nut foods. The majority of our people cannot obtain the nut preparations; few know how to prepare them properly for use, even if they could buy them. *(1901 Letter)*

370

*I*n grains, fruit, vegetables, and nuts are to be found all the food elements that we need. If we will come to the Lord in simplicity of mind, He will teach us how to prepare wholesome food free from the taint of flesh meat. *(Manuscript Files, 1906)*

371

The delicate organism of the body is worn out by the suicidal practices of those who ought to know better. *(Testimonies, Volume 2, 1868)*

372

All the food that is put into the stomach, from which the system cannot derive benefit, is a burden to nature in her work. It hinders the living machine. The system is clogged, and cannot successfully carry on its work. The vital organs are unnecessarily taxed, and the brain nerve power is called to the stomach to help the digestive organs carry on their work of disposing of an amount of food which does the system no good. *(Testimonies, Volume 2, 1870)*

"Significant alteration in the intestinal flora was observed when the patients changed from omnivorous to vegan diet. The fecal flora from patients with HI and LI differed significantly from each other at 1 and 13 months. This finding of an association between intestinal flora and disease activity may have implications for our understanding of how diet can affect rheumatoid arthritis."

British Journal of Rheumatology, 1994 Jul; 33(7):638–43

373

With nuts may be combined grains, fruits, and some roots, to make foods that are healthful and nourishing. Care should be taken, however, not to use too large a proportion of nuts. Those who realize ill effects from the use of nut foods may find the difficulty removed by attending to this precaution. *(Ministry of Healing, 1905)*

374

The digestive organs should never be burdened with a quantity or quality of food which it will tax the system to appropriate. All that is taken into the stomach, above what the system can use to convert into good blood, clogs the machinery; for it cannot be made into either flesh or blood, and its presence burdens the liver, and produces a morbid condition of the system. The stomach is overworked in its efforts to dispose of it, and then there is a sense of languor, which is interpreted to mean hunger, and without allowing the digestive organs time to rest from their severe labor, to recruit their energies, another immoderate amount is taken into the stomach, to set the weary machinery again in motion. The system receives less nourishment from too great a quantity of food, even of the right quality, than from a moderate quantity taken at regular periods. *(Testimonies, Volume 2, 1870)*

375

Nuts and nut foods are coming largely into use to take the place of flesh meats. *(Ministry of Healing, 1905)*

376

Careful attention should be given to the proper use of nut foods. Some kinds of nuts are not so wholesome as others. Do not reduce the bill of fare to a few articles composed largely of nut foods. These foods should not be used too freely. If they were used more sparingly by some, the results would be more satisfactory. As combined in large proportions with other articles in some of the recipes given, they make the food so rich that the system cannot properly assimilate it. *(1902 Letter)*

377

The oil in olives is a remedy for constipation and kidney diseases. *(1901 Letter)*

"It is the position of The American Dietetic Association (ADA) that appropriately planned vegetarian diets are healthful, are nutritionally adequate, and provide health benefits in the prevention and treatment of certain diseases."

Journal of the American Dietetic Association, November 1997, 97(1)

378

A fruit diet for a few days has often brought great relief to brain workers. Many times a short period of entire abstinence from food, followed by simple, moderate eating, has led to recovery through nature's own recuperative effort. An abstemious diet for a month or two would convince many sufferers that the path of self-denial is the path to health. *(Ministry of Healing, 1905)*

379

Nut foods should be made as inexpensive as possible, so that they can be procured by the poor. *(1901 Letter)*

380

I have been instructed that the nut foods are often used unwisely, that too large a proportion of nuts is used, that some nuts are not as wholesome as others. Almonds are preferable to peanuts; but peanuts, in limited quantities, may be used in connection with grains to make nourishing and digestible food. *(Testimonies, Volume 7, 1902)*

381

Υou place upon your tables butter, eggs, and meat, and your children partake of them. They are fed with the very things that will excite their animal passions, and then you come to meeting and ask God to bless and save your children. How high do your prayers go? You have a work to do first. When you have done all for your children which God has left for you to do, then you can with confidence claim the special help that God has promised to give you. *(Testimonies, Volume 2, 1870)*

"Many studies have tried to identify the one, single factor which makes the vegetarian diet beneficial for blood pressure, but the evidence so far shows that neither polyunsaturated fat, saturated fat, cholesterol, potassium, magnesium, sodium, or total protein intake are independently responsible for this effect. it is the totality of the vegetarian diet that is beneficial."

Canadian Journal of Physiology and Pharmacology, Jun 1986, 64 (6)

382

$\mathcal{V}$egetables, fruits, and grains should compose our diet. Not an ounce of flesh meat should enter our stomachs. *(Manuscript Files, 1903)*

383

$\mathcal{H}$ow can they take the life of God's creatures that they may consume the flesh as a luxury? Let them, rather, return to the wholesome and delicious food given to man in the beginning, and themselves practice, and teach their children to practice, mercy toward the dumb creatures that God has made and has placed under our dominion. *(Ministry of Healing, 1905)*

384

The eating of flesh is unnatural. We are to return to God's original purpose in the creation of man. *(Manuscript Files, 1903)*

385

Is it not time that all should aim to dispense with flesh foods? How can those who are seeking to become pure, refined, and holy, that they may have the companionship of heavenly angels, continue to use as food anything that has so harmful an effect on soul and body? *(Ministry of Healing, 1905)*

386

It was decided that at a certain camp meeting, cheese should not be sold to those on the ground; but on coming to the ground, Doctor Kellogg found to his surprise that a large quantity of cheese had been purchased for sale at the grocery. He and some others objected to this, but those in charge of the grocery said that they could not afford to lose the money invested in it. Upon this, Doctor Kellogg asked the price of the cheese, and bought the whole of it from them. He had traced the matter from cause to effect, and knew that some foods generally thought to be wholesome, were very injurious. *(1893 Letter)*

387

God demands that the appetite be cleansed, and that self-denial be practiced in regard to those things which are not good. This is a work that will have to be done before His people can stand before Him a perfected people. *(Testimonies, Volume 9, 1909)*

"High protein diets impair mental functioning."
International Journal of Obesity, Related Metabolic Disorders, 1995; 19:811

388

The moral evils of a flesh diet are not less marked than are the physical ills. Flesh food is injurious to health, and whatever affects the body has a corresponding effect on the mind and the soul. Think of the cruelty to animals that meat eating involves, and its effect on those who inflict and those who behold it. How it destroys the tenderness with which we should regard these creatures of God! *(Ministry of Healing, 1905)*

389

The unhealthful food placed in the stomach strengthens the appetites that war against the soul, developing the lower propensities. A diet of flesh meat tends to develop animalism. A development of animalism lessens spirituality, rendering the mind incapable of understanding truth. *(Review and Herald, May 27, 1902)*

390

The word of God plainly warns us that unless we abstain from fleshly lusts, the physical nature will be brought into conflict with the spiritual nature. Lustful eating wars against health and peace. Thus a warfare is instituted between the higher and the lower attributes of the man. The lower propensities, strong and active, oppress the soul. The highest interests of the being are imperiled by the indulgence of appetites unsanctioned by Heaven. *(Review and Herald, May 27, 1902)*

391

The common use of the flesh of dead animals has had a deteriorating influence upon the morals, as well as the physical institution. Ill health in a variety of forms, if effect could be traced to the cause, would reveal the sure result of flesh eating. *(Manuscript Files, 1887)*

392

The habits and practices of men have brought the earth into such a condition that some other food than animal food must be substituted for the human family. We do not need flesh food at all. God can give us something else. *(Australasian Union Conference Record, July 28, 1899*

"As modern young Japanese have adopted our ways of eating high amounts of fatty foods and more animal products, their age of onset of menses has gradually fallen over the last 50 years from 16 to 12.5 years."

Preventive Medicine, 1978; 7:205–17

393

Those who indulge in meat eating, tea drinking, and gluttony are sowing seeds for a harvest of pain and death. *(Review and Herald, May 27, 1902)*

394

Many times when meat is eaten, it decays in the stomach, and creates disease. Cancers, tumors, and pulmonary diseases are largely caused by meat eating. *(Pacific Union Recorder, October 9, 1902)*

395

Those who use flesh meat disregard all the warnings that God has given concerning this question. They have no evidence that they are walking in safe paths. They have not the slightest excuse for eating the flesh of dead animals. God's curse is resting upon the animal creation. *(Pacific Union Recorder, October 9, 1902)*

396

Could you know just the nature of the meat you eat, could you see the animals when living from which the flesh is taken when dead, you would turn with loathing from your flesh meats. *(Testimonies, Volume 2, 1870)*

397

The very animals whose flesh you eat, are frequently so diseased that, if left alone, they would die of themselves; but while the breath of life is in them, they are killed and brought to market. You take directly into your system humors and poison of the worst kind, and yet you realize it not. *(Testimonies, Volume 2, 1870)*

398

Often animals are taken to market and sold for food, when they are so diseased that their owners fear to keep them longer. And some of the processes of fattening them for market produce disease. Shut away from the light and pure air, breathing the atmosphere of filthy stables, perhaps fattening on decaying food, the entire body soon becomes contaminated with foul matter. *(Ministry of Healing, 1905)*

399

Flesh was never the best food; but its use is now doubly objectionable, since disease in animals is so rapidly increasing. *(Ministry of Healing, 1905)*

"Researchers followed 384 men with prostate cancer over a five-year period . . . those who consumed the most saturated fat—the kind particularly prevalent in meats and dairy products—had three times the risk of dying from the disease, compared to those with the lowest saturated fat intake."

European Journal of Urology, 1999; 388:91

400

Very many animals are sold for the city market known to be diseased by those who have sold them, and those who buy them are not always ignorant of the matter. Especially in larger cities this is practiced to a great extent, and meat eaters know not that they are eating diseased animals. *(Spiritual Gifts, Book 4, 1864)*

401

Many die of disease caused wholly by meat eating; yet the world does not seem to be the wiser. Animals are frequently killed that have been driven quite a distance for the slaughter. Their blood has become heated. They are full of flesh, and have been deprived of healthy exercise, and when they have to travel far, they become surfeited and exhausted, and in that condition are killed for market. Their blood is highly inflamed, and those who eat of their meat, eat poison. Some are not immediately affected, while others are attacked with severe pain, and die from fever, cholera, or some unknown disease. *(Spiritual Gifts, Book 4, 1864)*

402

Worldly physicians cannot account for the rapid increase of disease among the human family. But we know that much of this suffering is caused by the eating of dead flesh. The animals are diseased, and by partaking of their flesh, we plant the seeds of disease in our own tissue and blood. Then when exposed to the changes in a malarious atmosphere, these are more sensibly felt; also when we are exposed to prevailing epidemics and contagious diseases, the system is not in a condition to resist the disease. *(1901 Letter)*

403

You have flesh, but it is not good material. You are worse off for this amount of flesh. If you would each come down to a more spare diet, which would take from you twenty-five or thirty pounds of your gross flesh, you should be much less liable to disease. The eating of flesh meats has made a poor quality of blood and flesh. Your systems are in a state of inflammation, prepared to take on disease. You are liable to acute attacks of disease, and to sudden death, because you do not possess the strength of constitution to rally and resist disease. There will come a time when the strength and health you have flattered yourself you possessed will prove to be weakness. *(Testimonies, Volume 2, 1868)*

"Evidence strongly suggests that a high intake of plant-based foods, and a low intake of animal products contributes to the excellent health of Mediterranean populations. The high consumption of red meat in Western diets is associated with increased risks of heart disease, some cancers, and urinary calcium losses likely to contribute to osteoporosis."

American Journal of Clinical Nutrition, 1995; 61, 1416

404

Some animals that are brought to the slaughter seem to realize by instinct what is to take place, and they become furious, and literally mad. They are killed while in that state, and their flesh is prepared for market. Their meat is poison, and has produced, in those who have eaten it, cramps, convulsions, apoplexy, and sudden death. Yet the cause of all this suffering is not attributed to the meat. *(Testimonies, Volume 2, 1868)*

405

Animals are often transported long distances and subjected to great suffering in reaching a market. Taken from the green pastures and traveling for weary miles over the hot, dusty roads, or crowded into filthy cars, feverish and exhausted, often for many hours deprived of food and water, the poor creatures are driven to their death, that human beings may feast on the carcasses. *(Ministry of Healing, 1905)*

406

The liability to take disease is increased tenfold by meat eating. *(Testimonies, Volume 2, 1868)*

407

Cancers, tumors, and all inflammatory diseases are largely caused by meat eating. From the light God has given me, the prevalence of cancer and tumors is largely due to gross living on dead flesh. *(Excerpts From Unpublished Testimonies in Regard to Flesh Foods, 1896)*

> "Cancer induction can be decreased by avoiding the formation of carcinogens, reducing their metabolic activation, or increasing their detoxification. Excessive dietary salt, and heterocyclic arylamines formed in cooking of meats or fish, and high intake of 40% of calories in fats are health risks, but vegetables, fruits, tea, soy products, and fibers are protective."
>
> *Biofactors*, 2000, Vol. 12, p73

408

Flesh meats will depreciate the blood. Cook meat with spices, and eat it with rich cakes and pies, and you have a bad quality of blood. The system is too heavily taxed in disposing of this kind of food. *(Testimonies, Volume 2, 1870)*

409

The testimony of examiners is that very few animals are free from disease, and that the practice of eating largely of meat is contracting diseases of all kinds,—cancers, tumors, scrofula, tuberculosis, and numbers of other like affections. *(Manuscript Files, 1897)*

410

Some animals are inhumanly treated while being brought to the slaughter. They are literally tortured, and after they have endured many hours of extreme suffering, are butchered. Swine have been prepared for market even while the plague was upon them, and their poisonous flesh has spread contagious diseases, and great mortality has followed. *(Spiritual Gifts, Book 4, 1864)*

411

The meat diet is the serious question. Shall human beings live on the flesh of dead animals? The answer, from the light that God has given is, No, decidedly No. Health reform institutions should educate on this question. Physicians who claim to understand the human organism ought not to encourage their patients to subsist on the flesh of dead animals. They should point out the increase of disease in the animal kingdom. *(Manuscript Files, 1897)*

412

Those who use flesh foods little know what they are eating. Often if they could see the animals when living and know the quality of the meat they eat, they would turn from it with loathing. People are continually eating flesh that is filled with tuberculosis and cancerous germs. Tuberculosis, cancer, and other fatal diseases are thus communicated. *(Ministry of Healing, 1905)*

"Vegan diets are appropriate for all stages of the life cycle, including during pregnancy and lactation."

American Journal of Clinical Nutrition, 1994; 59 (suppl):1176S–1181S

413

Flesh meats constitute the principle article of food upon the tables of some families, until their blood is filled with cancerous and scrofulous humors. Their bodies are composed of what they eat. But when suffering and disease come upon them, it is considered an affliction of Providence. *(Testimonies, Volume 3, 1905)*

414

I have felt urged by the Spirit of God to set before several the fact that their suffering and ill health was caused by a disregard of the light given them upon health reform. I have shown them that their meat diet, which was supposed to be essential, was not necessary, and that, as they were composed of what they ate, brain, bone, and muscle were in an unwholesome condition, because they lived on the flesh of dead animals; that their blood was being corrupted by this improper diet; that the flesh which they ate was diseased, and their entire system was becoming gross and corrupted. *(Excerpts From Unpublished Testimonies in Regard to Flesh Foods, 1896)*

415

*T*hose who use flesh meats freely, do not always have an unclouded brain and an active intellect, because the use of the flesh of animals tends to cause a grossness of body, and to benumb the finer sensibilities of the mind. *(Christian Temperance and Bible Hygiene, 1890)*

416

*N*either study nor violent exercise should be engaged in immediately after a full meal; this would be a violation of the laws of the system. Immediately after eating there is a strong draft upon the nervous energy. The brain force is called into active exercise to assist the stomach; therefore, when the mind or body is taxed heavily after eating, the process of digestion is hindered. The vitality of the system, which is needed to carry on the work in one direction, is called away and set to work in another. *(Testimonies, Volume 2, 1870)*

417

I was instructed that the use of flesh meat has a tendency to animalize the nature, and to rob men and women of the love and sympathy which they should feel for every one. *(Manuscript Files, 1904)*

"A diet enriched with fruit, vegetables, nuts, whole grains and mustard or soy bean oil is associated with a pronounced decline in coronary artery disease morbidity and mortality. The long-term benefits may be even more substantial."

The Lancet, 2002; 360:1455–1461

418

*T*he effect of cheese is deleterious. Fine-flour bread does not impart to the system the nourishment that is to be found in unbolted-wheat bread. Its common use will not keep the system in the best condition. *(Christian Temperance and Bible Hygiene, 1890)*

419

A meat diet changes the disposition and strengthens animalism. We are composed of what we eat, and eating much flesh will diminish intellectual activity. Students would accomplish much more in their studies if they never tasted meat. When the animal part of the human agent is strengthened by meat eating, the intellectual powers diminish proportionately. A religious life can be more successfully gained and maintained if meat is discarded, for this diet stimulates into intense activity lustful propensities, and enfeebles the moral and spiritual nature. "The flesh warreth against the spirit, and the spirit against the flesh." *(Excerpts From Unpublished Testimonies in Regard to Flesh Foods, 1896)*

420

There is an alarming lethargy shown on the subject of unconscious sensualism. It is customary to eat the flesh of dead animals. This stimulates the lower passions of the human organism. *(Excerpts From Unpublished Testimonies in Regard to Flesh Foods, 1896)*

421

There are many kinds of wholesome food. But we do say that flesh meat is not the right food for God's people. It animalizes human beings. In a country such as this, where there are fruits, grains, and nuts in abundance, how can one think that he must eat the flesh of dead animals? *(Manuscript Files, 1904)*

422

Your family have partaken largely of flesh meats, and the animal propensities have been strengthened, while the intellectual have been weakened. We are composed of what we eat, and if we subsist largely upon the flesh of dead animals, we shall partake of their nature. You have encouraged the grosser part of your organization, while the more refined has been weakened. *(Testimonies, Volume 2, 1868)*

423

The intellectual, the moral, and the physical powers are depreciated by the habitual use of flesh meats. Meat eating deranges the system, beclouds the intellect, and blunts the moral sensibilities. We say to you, dear brother and sister, your safest course is to let meat alone. *(Testimonies, Volume 2, 1868)*

"Vegetarians have a lower incidence of hypertension than non vegetarians."

American Journal of Clinical Nutrition, 1994; 59 (suppl)

424

The effects of a flesh diet may not be immediately realized; but this is no evidence that it is not harmful. Few can be made to believe that it is the meat they have eaten which has poisoned their blood and caused their suffering. *(Ministry of Healing, 1905)*

425

The eating of pork has produced scrofula, leprosy, and cancerous humors. Pork eating is still causing the most intense suffering to the human race. *(How to Live, Book 1, 1865)*

426

We have plenty of good things to satisfy hunger without bringing corpses upon our table to compose our bill of fare. *(Excerpts From Unpublished Testimonies in Regard to Flesh Foods, 1890)*

427

Many die of diseases wholly due to meat eating, when the real cause is scarcely suspected by themselves or others. Some do not immediately feel its effects, but this is no evidence that it does not hurt them. It may be doing its work surely upon the system, yet for the time being the victim may realize nothing of it. *(Christian Temperance and Bible Hygiene, 1890)*

428

You have repeatedly said in defense of your indulgence of meat eating, "However injurious it may be to others, it does not injure me, for I have used it all my life." But you know not how well you might have been if you had abstained from the use of flesh meats. *(Testimonies, Volume 2, 1868)*

> "I don't understand why asking people to eat a well-balanced vegetarian diet is considered drastic, while it is medically conservative to cut people open or put them on powerful cholesterol-lowering drugs for the rest of their lives."
>
> Dean Ornish, M.D.

429

I have the subject presented to me in different aspects. The mortality caused by meat eating is not discerned; if it were, we would hear no more arguments and excuses in favor of the indulgence of the appetite for dead flesh. *(Excerpts From Unpublished Testimonies in Regard to Flesh Foods, 1896)*

430

Pork, although one of the most common articles of diet, is one of the most injurious. God did not prohibit the Hebrews from eating swine's flesh merely to show His authority, but because it was not a proper article of food for man. It would fill the system with scrofula, and especially in that warm climate produced leprosy, and disease of various kinds. Its influence upon the system in that climate was far more injurious than in a colder climate. But God never designed the swine to be eaten under any circumstances. *(How to Love, Book 1, 1865)*

431

God has given you light and knowledge, which you have professed to believe came direct from Him, instructing you to deny appetite. You know that the use of swine's flesh is contrary to His express command, given not because He wished to especially show His authority, but because it would be injurious to those who should eat it. Its use would cause the blood to become impure, so that scrofula and other humors would corrupt the system, and the whole organism would suffer. Especially would the fine, sensitive nerves of the brain become enfeebled and so beclouded that sacred things would not be discerned, but be placed upon the low level with common things. *(Testimonies, Volume 2, 1868)*

432

It is not the physical health alone which is injured by pork eating. The mind is affected, and the finer sensibilities are blunted by the use of this gross article of food. It is impossible for the flesh of any living creatures to be healthy when filth is their natural element, and when they will feed upon every detestable thing. The flesh of swine is composed of what they eat. If human beings eat their flesh, their blood and their flesh will be corrupted by impurities conveyed to them through the swine. *(How to Live, Book 1, 1865)*

"Mortality rates are similar or lower for vegetarians than for nonvegetarians. Data are strong that vegetarians are at lesser risk for obesity, atonic constipation, lung cancer, and alcoholism. Evidence is good that risks for hypertension, coronary artery disease, type II diabetes, and gallstones are lower."

American Journal of Clinical Nutrition, 1988 Sep; 48 (3 Suppl):712–38

433

The tissues of the swine swarm with parasites. Of the swine, God said, "It is unclean unto you; ye shall not eat of their flesh, nor touch their dead carcass." This command was given because swine's flesh is unfit for food. Swine are scavengers, and this is the only use they were intended to serve. Never, under any circumstances, was their flesh to be eaten by human beings. *(Ministry of Healing, 1905)*

434

The heathen used pork as an article of food, and American people have used pork freely as an important article of diet. Swine's flesh would not be palatable to the taste in its natural state. It is made agreeable to the appetite by high seasoning, which makes a very bad thing worse. Swine's flesh above all other flesh meats, produces a bad state of the blood. Those who eat freely of pork can but be diseased. Those who have much outdoor exercise do not realize the bad effects of pork eating, as those do whose life is mostly indoors, and whose habits are sedentary, and whose labor is mental. *(How to Live, Book 1, 1865)*

435

In many places fish become so contaminated by the filth on which they feed as to be a cause of disease. This is especially the case where the fish come in contact with the sewage of large cities. The fish that are fed on the contents of the drains may pass into distant waters, and may be caught where the water is pure and fresh. Thus when used as food they bring disease and death on those who do not suspect the danger. *(Ministry of Healing, 1905)*

"84 prostate cancer men who were able to defer treatment because of a careful watch on their prostate-specific antigen (PSA) participated in the study. Half the men were assigned to usual care (control group) and the remaining half to a low-fat, vegan diet, along with regular exercice and stress management. In the control group, the PSA levels rose over the three-month study period, and 7 required additional treatment. But in the 42 men assigned to the vegan diet and lifestyle intervention, the average PSA level dropped from 6.3 to 5.8, and none required further treatment."

Urology, 2001; 57 (4 Suppl 1):200–1

436

The meat is served reeking with fat, because it suits the perverted taste. Both the blood and the fat of animals are consumed as a luxury. But the Lord gave special directions that these should not be eaten. Why? Because their use would make a diseased current of blood in the human system. The disregard for the Lord's special directions has brought a variety of difficulties and diseases upon human beings. *(1890 Letter)*

437

The more largely flesh composes the diet of teachers and pupils, the less susceptible will be the mind to comprehend spiritual things. The animal propensities are strengthened, and the fine sensibilities of the mind are blunted. Diligent study is not the principal cause of the breaking down of the mental powers. The main cause is improper diet, irregular meals, and a lack of physical exercise. Irregular hours for eating and sleeping sap the brain forces. *(Youth's Instructor, May 31, 1894)*

"Scientific data suggest positive relationships between a vegetarian diet and reduced risk for several chronic degenerative diseases and conditions, including obesity, coronary artery disease, hypertension, diabetes mellitus, and some types of cancer."

Journal of the American Dietetic Association, November 1997, 97(1)

438

Some will find it as difficult to leave off flesh eating as it is for the drunkard to give up his dram; but they will be the better for the change. *(Ministry of Healing, 1905)*

439

The smell of the raw flesh is offensive to all whose senses have not been depraved by culture of the unnatural appetites. What more unpleasant sight to a reflective mind than the beasts slain to be devoured? If the light God has given in regard to health reform is disregarded, He will not work a miracle to keep in health those who pursue a course to make themselves sick. *(Excerpts From Unpublished Testimonies in Regard to Flesh Foods, 1896)*

440

The diet of the animals is vegetables and grains. Must the vegetables be animalized, must they be incorporated into the system of animals, before we get them? Must we obtain our vegetable diet by eating the flesh of dead creatures? He gave to Adam charge of the garden, to dress it, and to care for it, saying, "To you it shall be for meat." One animal was not to destroy another animal for food. *(1896 Letter)*

441

The grains, with fruits, nuts, and vegetables, contain all the nutritive properties necessary to make good blood. These elements are not so well or fully supplied by a flesh diet. Had the use of flesh been essential to health and strength, animal food would have been included in the diet appointed man in the beginning. *(Ministry of Healing, 1905)*

442

The inquiry with many is, What shall I eat, and how shall I live, to best enjoy the present time? Duty and principle are laid aside for present gratification. If we would have health, we must live for it. If we perfect Christian character, we must live for it. Parents are, in a great degree, responsible for the physical health and morals of their children. They should instruct their children and urge them to conform to the laws of health for their own sake, to save themselves unhappiness and suffering. How strange that mothers should indulge their children to the ruin of their physical, mental, and moral health! What can be the character of such fondness! These mothers make their children unfit for happiness in this life, and render the prospect of the future life very uncertain. *(Health Reformer, December, 1870)*

443

Flesh food also is harmful. Its naturally stimulating effect should be a sufficient argument against its use; and the almost universally diseased condition of animals makes it doubly objectionable. It tends to irritate the nerves and to excite the passions, thus giving the balance of power to the lower propensities. *(Education, 1903)*

444

*I*t is not necessary to take the life of any of God's creatures to supply our ordinary needs. *(Christian Temperance and Bible Hygiene, 1890)*

445

*W*hen flesh is discarded, its place should be supplied with a variety of grains, nuts, vegetables, and fruits, that will be both nourishing and appetizing. This is especially necessary in the case of those who are weak, or who are taxed with continuous labor. In some countries, where poverty abounds, flesh is the cheapest food. Under these circumstances, the change will be made with greater difficulty; but it can be effected. We should, however, consider the situation of the people and the power of lifelong habit, and should be careful not to urge even right ideas unduly. None should be urged to make the change abruptly. *(Ministry of Healing, 1905)*

"In reality, cow's milk, especially processed cow's milk, has been linked to a variety of health problems, including: mucous production, hemoglobin loss, childhood diabetes, heart disease, atherosclerosis, arthritis, kidney stones, mood swings, depression, irritability, and allergies."

Townsend Medical Letter, May 1995; Julie Klotter, MD

446

*W*ith care and skill, dishes may be prepared that will be both nutritious and appetizing, and will, to a great degree, take the place of flesh food. In all cases, educate the conscience, enlist the will, supply good, wholesome food, and the change will be readily made, and the demand for flesh will soon cease. *(Ministry of Healing, 1905)*

447

Those who are in a position where it is possible to secure a vegetarian diet, but who choose to follow their own preferences in this matter, eating and drinking as they please, will gradually grow careless of the instruction the Lord has given regarding other phases of the present truth, and will lose their perception of what is truth; they will surely reap as they have sown. *(Testimonies, Volume 9, 1909)*

448

The proper cooking of foods is a most important accomplishment. Especially where meat is not made a principal article of food is good cooking an essential requirement. Something must be prepared to take the place of meat, and these substitutes for meat must be well prepared, so that meat will not be desired. *(1896 Letter)*

449

While we do not make the use of flesh meat a test, while we do not want to force any one to give up its use, yet it is our duty to request that no minister of the conference shall make light of or oppose the message of reform on this point. If, in the face of the light God has given concerning the effect of meat eating on the system, you will still continue to eat meat, you must bear the consequences. *(1902 Letter)*

"Vegetarian diets offer disease protection benefits because higher concentration of antioxidants such as vitamins C and E, carotenoids, and phytochemicals."

American Journal of Clinical Nutrition, 1996; 63 (suppl)

450

For more than forty years I have eaten but two meals a day. And if I have a specially important work to do, I limit the quantity of food that I take. I regard it as my duty to refuse to place in my stomach any food that I have reason to believe will create disorder. *(1908 Letter)*

451

Hot biscuits and flesh meats are entirely out of harmony with health reform principles. If we would allow reason to take the place of impulse and love of sensual indulgence, we should not taste of the flesh of dead animals. *(Excerpts From Unpublished Testimonies in Regard to Flesh Foods, 1896)*

452

Hot biscuits and flesh meats are entirely out of harmony with health reform principles. If we would allow reason to take the place of impulse and love of sensual indulgence, we should not taste of the flesh of dead animals. *(Excerpts From Unpublished Testimonies in Regard to Flesh Foods, 1896)*

453

I have been instructed that flesh food has a tendency to animalize the nature, to rob men and women of that love and sympathy which they should feel for every one, and to give the lower passions control over the higher powers of the being. If meat eating were ever healthful, it is not safe now. Cancers, tumors, and pulmonary diseases are largely caused by meat eating. *(Testimonies, Volume 9, 1909)*

454

$\mathcal{N}$ever be ashamed to say, "No, thank you; I do not eat meat. I have conscientious scruples against eating the flesh of dead animals." If tea is offered, refuse it, giving your reason for so doing. Explain that it is harmful, and though stimulating for a time, the stimulus soon wears off, and a corresponding depression is felt. *(Manuscript Files, 1901)*

> "Some plant proteins may increase survival rates and decrease proteinuria, glomerular filtration rate, renal blood flow, and histologic renal damage compared with a non vegetarian diet."
>
> *Clinical Nutrition,* 1995; 10

455

$\mathcal{I}f$ we could be benefited by indulging the desire for flesh foods, I would not make this appeal to you; but I know we cannot. Flesh foods are injurious to the physical well-being, and we should learn to do without them. *(Testimonies, Volume 9, 1909)*

456

$\mathcal{M}$any parents act as if they were bereft of reason. They are in a state of lethargy, palsied by the indulgence of perverted appetite and debasing passion. *(Manuscript Files, 1902)*

457

$\mathcal{T}$he appetite will be much better if changes in the food are made. Be uniform. Do not have several kinds of food on the table at one meal, and no variety the next. Study economy in this line. *(1884 Letter)*

458

I have been instructed that the students in our schools are not to be served with flesh foods or with food preparations that are known to be unhealthful. Nothing that will serve to encourage a desire for stimulants should be placed on the tables. *(Testimonies, Volume 9, 1909)*

459

*S*ubsisting on the flesh of dead animals is a gross way of living, and as a people, we should be working a change, a reform, teaching the people that there are healthful preparations of food that will give them more strength, and better preserve their health, than meat. *(1884 Letter)*

460

*T*he sin of this age is gluttony in eating and drinking. Indulgence of appetite is the God which many worship. Those who are connected with the Health Institute should set a right example in these things. They should move conscientiously in the fear of God, and not be controlled by a perverted taste. They should be thoroughly enlightened in regard to the principles of health reform, and under all circumstances should stand under its banner. *(1884 Letter)*

"Tufts University researchers interviewed more than 900 men and women aged 69 to 93 about their diets and measured their bone density at several skeletal sites. Men who consumed the most fruit, vegetables and cereal had denser bones and women who ate a great deal of candy had the lowest bone mineral density."

American Journal of Clinical Nutrition, 2002; 76:245–52

461

$\mathcal{A}$ positive injury is done to the system by continuous meat eating. There is no excuse for it but a depraved, perverted appetite. You may ask, Would you do away entirely with meat eating? I answer, It will eventually come to this, but we are not prepared for this step just now. Meat eating will eventually be done away. The flesh of animals will no longer compose a part of our diet; and we shall look upon a butcher's shop with disgust. *(1884 Letter)*

462

$\mathcal{W}$e are built up from that which we eat. Shall we strengthen the animal passions by eating animal food? In the place of educating the taste to love this gross diet, it is high time that we were educating ourselves to subsist upon fruits, grains, and vegetables. This is the work of all who are connected with our institutions. Use less and less meat, until it is not used at all. *(1884 Letter)*

463

$\mathcal{C}$offee is a hurtful indulgence. It temporarily excites the mind to unwonted action, but the aftereffect is exhaustion, prostration, paralysis of the mental, moral, and physical powers. The mind becomes enervated, and unless through determined effort the habit is overcome, the activity of the brain is permanently lessened. All these nerve irritants are wearing away the life forces, and the restlessness caused by shattered nerves, the impatience, the mental feebleness, become a warring element, antagonizing to spiritual progress. *(Christian Temperance and Bible Hygiene, 1890)*

464

$\mathcal{B}$ecause of meat eating, many die, and they do not understand the cause. If the truth were known, it would bear testimony it was the flesh of animals that have passed through death. The thought of feeding on dead flesh is repulsive, but there is something besides this. In eating meat we partake of diseased dead flesh, and this sows its seed of corruption in the human organism. *(1898 Letter)*

"Vegetarians tend to have a lower incidence of hypertension than non-vegetarians. This effect appears to be independent of both body weight and sodium intake."

American Journal of Clinical Nutrition, 1994; 59 (supplement):1130–1135

465

$\mathcal{T}$hen the fact that meat is largely diseased, should lead us to make strenuous efforts to discontinue its use entirely. My position now is to let meat altogether alone. It will be hard for some to do this, as hard as for the rum drinker to forsake his dram; but they will be better for the change. *(1898 Letter)*

466

$\mathcal{F}$ood should not be washed down; no drink is needed with meals. Eat slowly, and allow the saliva to mingle with the food. Do not eat largely of salt; give up bottled pickles; keep fiery spiced food out of your stomach; eat fruit with your meals, and the irritation which calls for so much drink will cease to exist. But if anything is needed to quench thirst, pure water, drunk some little time before or after the meal, is all that nature requires. *(Review and Herald, July 29, 1884)*

467

When meat is not used as it has been, you will learn a more correct way of cooking, and will be able to supply the place of meat with something else. Many healthful dishes can be prepared which are free from grease and from the flesh of dead animals. A variety of simple dishes, perfectly healthful and nourishing, may be provided, aside from meat. Hearty men must have plenty of vegetables, fruits, and grains. *(1884 Letter)*

468

The disease upon animals is becoming more and more common, and our only safety now is in leaving meat entirely alone. The most aggravated diseases are now prevalent, and the very last thing that physicians who are enlightened should do, is to advise patients to eat meat. *(1898 Letter)*

"Evidence suggests that most of the chronic degenerative diseases can be reversed or at least suspended from further development, by consuming a plant-based diet. This diet has a comprehensive ability to control the expression of the genes that predispose to many diseases such as heart disease, cancer, diabetes, obesity, childhood allergies. The beneficial effects of consuming a plant-based diet can only be fully appreciated and demonstrated when it is understood that nutrients work in concert."

T. Colin Campbell, Ph.D. Cornell University, "The China Study"

469

Disease is contracted by the use of meat. The diseased flesh of these dead carcasses is sold in the market places, and disease among men is the sure result. *(1898 Letter)*

470

$\mathcal{M}$eat eating should not come into the prescription for any invalids from any physicians from among those who understand these things. Disease in cattle is making meat eating a dangerous matter. The Lord's curse is upon the earth, upon man, upon beasts, upon the fish in the sea; and as transgression becomes almost universal, the curse will be permitted to become as broad and as deep as the transgression. *(1898 Letter)*

471

$\mathcal{Y}$ou may think you cannot work without meat. I thought so once, but I know that in His original plan, God did not provide for the flesh of dead animals to compose the diet for man. It is a gross, perverted taste that will accept such food. *(1884 Letter)*

472

$\mathcal{M}$any make a mistake in drinking cold water with their meals. Taken with meals, water diminishes the flow of the salivary glands; and the colder the water, the greater the injury to the stomach. Ice water or ice lemonade, drunk with meals, will arrest digestion until the system has imparted sufficient warmth to the stomach to enable it to take up its work again. *(Review and Herald, July 29, 1884)*

473

$\mathcal{T}$he stimulating diet and drink of this day are not conducive to the best state of health. Tea, coffee, and tobacco are all stimulating, and contain poisons. *(Review and Herald, February 21, 1888)*

474

$\mathcal{T}$ea is poisonous to the system. Tea and coffee drinkers carry the marks upon their faces. The skin becomes sallow, and assumes a lifeless appearance. The glow of health is not seen upon the countenance. *(Testimonies, Volume 2, 1868)*

"The association between vegetarianism and blood pressure was studied in relation to obesity, sex and aspects of lifestyle. There is an additional blood pressure reducing effect associated with a vegetarian diet."

Clinical Experimental Pharmacology and Physiology, May 1982, 327–30

475

$\mathcal{G}$od gave man no permission to eat animal food until after the flood. Everything had been destroyed upon which man could subsist, and therefore the Lord in their necessity gave Noah permission to eat of the clean animals which he had taken with him into the ark. But animal food was not the most healthful article of food for man. *(Spiritual Gifts, Book 4, 1890)*

476

$\mathcal{I}$ was somewhat surprised at your argument as to why a meat-eating diet kept you in strength, for, if you put yourself out of the question, your reason will teach you that a meat diet is not of as much advantage as you suppose. You know how you would answer a tobacco devotee if he urged, as a plea for the use of tobacco, the arguments you have advanced as a reason why you should continue the use of the flesh of dead animals as food. *(1896 Letter)*

477

Tea acts as a stimulant, and, to a certain extent, produces intoxication. The action of coffee and many other popular drinks is similar. The first effect is exhilarating. The nerves of the stomach are excited; these convey irritation to the brain, and this in turn is aroused to impart increased action to the heart, and short-lived energy to the entire system. Fatigue is forgotten, the strength seems to be increased. The intellect is aroused, the imagination becomes more vivid. Because of these results, many suppose that their tea or coffee is doing them great good. But this is a mistake. Tea and coffee do not nourish the system. Their effect is produced before there has been time for digestion and assimilation, and what seems to be strength is only nervous excitement. When the influence of the stimulant is gone, the unnatural force abates, and the result is a corresponding degree of languor and debility. *(Ministry of Healing, 1905)*

478

Tea, coffee, and tobacco, as well as alcoholic drinks, are different degrees in the scale of artificial stimulants. The effect of tea and coffee, as heretofore shown, tends in the same direction as that of wine and cider, liquor and tobacco. *(Christian Temperance and Bible Hygiene, 1890)*

479

Cheese should never be introduced into the stomach. Butter is less harmful when eaten on cold bread than when used in cooking; but, as a rule, it is better to dispense with it altogether. Cheese is still more objectionable; it is wholly unfit for food. *(Ministry of Healing, 1905)*

480

The animal creation is diseased, and it is difficult to determine the amount of disease in the human family that is the result of meat eating. We read constantly in the daily papers about the inspection of meat. Butcher shops are continually being cleaned out; the meat being sold is condemned as unfit for use. *(1898 Letter)*

"Every 12 minutes someone dies from breast cancer. Yet women who eat as few as two servings of vegetables per day reduce their breast cancer risk by 30%."
Annals of the New York Academy of Sciences, 768 (Sept. 30, 1995): 1–11

481

Poor cooking produces disease and bad tempers; the system becomes deranged, and heavenly things cannot be discerned. There is more religion in good cooking than you have any idea of. When I have been away from home sometimes, I have known that the bread upon the table, as well as most of the other food, would hurt me; but I would be obliged to eat a little in order to sustain life. It is a sin in the sight of Heaven to have such food. *(Christian Temperance and Bible Hygiene, 1890)*

482

Diseases of every stripe and type have been brought upon human beings by the use of tea and coffee and the narcotics, opium and tobacco. These hurtful indulgences must be given up, not only one but all; for all are hurtful, and ruinous to the physical, mental, and moral powers, and should be discontinued from a health standpoint. *(Manuscript Files, 1887)*

483

When a physician sees that a patient is suffering from an ailment caused by improper eating and drinking, yet neglects to tell him of this, and to point out the need of reform, he is doing a fellow being an injury. Drunkards, maniacs, those who are given over to licentiousness,—all appeal to the physician to declare clearly and distinctly that suffering is the result of sin. We have received great light on health reform. Why, then, are we not more decidedly in earnest in striving to counteract the causes that produce disease? Seeing the continual conflict with pain, laboring constantly to alleviate suffering, how can our physicians hold their peace? Can they refrain from lifting the voice in warning? Are they benevolent and merciful if they do not teach strict temperance as a remedy for disease? *(Testimonies, Volume 7, 1902)*

484

A great amount of good can be done by enlightening all to whom we have access, as to the best means, not only of curing the sick, but of preventing disease and suffering. The physician who endeavors to enlighten his patients as to the nature and causes of their maladies and to teach them how to avoid disease, may have uphill work; but if he is a conscientious reformer, he will talk plainly of the ruinous effects of self-indulgence in eating, drinking, and dressing, of the over-taxation of the vital forces that has brought his patients where they are. He will not increase the evil by administering drugs till exhausted nature gives up the struggle, but will teach the patients how to form correct habits, and to aid nature in her work of restoration by a wise use of her own simple remedies. *(Christian Temperance and Bible Hygiene, 1890)*

485

*N*ever take tea, coffee, beer, wine, or any spirituous liquors. Water is the best liquid possible to cleanse the tissues. *(Review and Herald, July 29, 1884)*

486

*M*ake fruit the article of diet to be placed on your table, which shall constitute the bill of fare. The juices of fruit, mingled with bread, will be highly enjoyed. Good, ripe, un-decayed fruit is a thing we should thank the Lord for, because it is beneficial to health. *(1896 Letter)*

487

*W*e should educate ourselves, not only to live in harmony with the laws of health, but to teach others the better way. Many, even of those who profess to believe the special truths for this time, are lamentably ignorant with regard to health and temperance. They need to be educated, line upon line, precept upon precept. The subject must be kept fresh before them. This matter must not be passed over as non-essential; for nearly every family needs to be stirred up on the question. The conscience must be aroused to the duty of practicing the principles of true reform. *(Christian Temperance and Bible Hygiene, 1890)*

"A lipid-lowering portfolio containing vegetable proteins, especially soy, plant sterols an high fiber intakes combined with low saturated and trans fatty acids and cholesterol, would go a long way to reducing serum lipids and coronary heart disease risk seen in the modern Western diet."

Asia Pacific Journal of Clinical Nutrition, October 2002; 9,3

488

*I*n all our missions, women of intelligence should have charge of the domestic arrangements,—women who know how to prepare food nicely and healthfully. The table should be abundantly supplied with food of the best quality. *(Christian Temperance and Bible Hygiene, 1890)*

"A well-planned vegetarian diet may be useful in the prevention and treatment of renal disease . . . plant proteins may increase survival rates and decrease proteinuria, glomerular filtration rate, renal blood flow, and histologic renal damage compared with a nonvegetarian diet."

Journal of the American Dietetic Association, November 1997; 97(1) citing *Nephronology,* 1996; 74:390–394

489

*T*here should be more earnest efforts made to enlighten the people upon the great subject of health reform. Tracts of four, eight, twelve, sixteen, and more pages, containing pointed, well-written articles on this great question, should be scattered like the leaves of autumn. *(Review and Herald, November 4, 1875)*

490

*C*ooking schools are to be held. The people are to be taught how to prepare wholesome food. They are to be shown the need of discarding unhealthful foods. But we should never advocate a starvation diet. It is possible to have a wholesome, nutritious diet without the use of tea, coffee, and flesh food. The work of teaching the people how to prepare a dietary that is at once wholesome and appetizing, is of the utmost importance. *(Testimonies, Volume 9, 1909)*

"In addition to the health advantages, other considerations that may lead a person to adopt a vegetarian diet pattern include concern for the environment, ecology, and world hunger issues. Vegetarians also cite economic reasons, ethical considerations, and religious beliefs."

Journal of the American Dietetic Association, November 1997; 97

491

*A*ll should have the light on this question, but let it be carefully presented. Habits that have been thought right for a lifetime are not to be changed by harsh or hasty measures. We should educate the people at our camp meetings and other large gatherings. While the principles of health reform should be presented, let the teaching be backed by example. Let no meat be found at our restaurants or dining tents, but let its place be supplied with fruits, grains, and vegetables. We must practice what we teach. When sitting at a table where meat is provided, we are not to make a raid upon those who use it, but we should let it alone ourselves, and when asked our reasons for doing this, we should in a kindly manner explain why we do not use it.
(1896 Letter)

492

*S*ome, after adopting a vegetarian diet, return to the use of flesh meat. This is foolish, indeed, and reveals a lack of knowledge of how to provide proper food in the place of meat. Cooking schools, conducted by wise instructors, are to be held in America and in other lands. Everything that we can do should be done to show the people the value of the reform diet.
(Testimonies, Volume 7, 1902)

493

$\mathcal{E}$very hygienic restaurant should be a school for the workers connected with it. In the cities this line of work may be done on a much larger scale than in smaller places. But in every place where there is a church and a church school, instruction should be given in regard to the preparation of simple health foods for the use of those who wish to live in accordance with the principles of health reform. And in all our missionary fields a similar work can be done. The work of combining fruits, seeds, grains, and roots into wholesome foods, is the Lord's work. In every place where a church has been established, let the church members walk humbly before God. Let them seek to enlighten the people with health reform principles. *(Manuscript Files, 1900)*

494

In all our schools there should be those who are fitted to teach cooking. Classes for instruction in this subject should be held. Those who are receiving a training for service suffer a great loss when they do not gain a knowledge of how to prepare food so that it is both wholesome and palatable. *(Counsels to Teachers, 1913)*

495

$\mathcal{G}$reater efforts should be put forth to educate the people in the principles of health reform. Cooking schools should be established, and house-to-house instruction should be given in the art of cooking wholesome food. Old and young should learn how to cook more simply. Wherever the truth is presented, the people are to be taught how to prepare food in a simple, yet appetizing way. They are to be shown that a nourishing diet can be provided without the use of flesh foods. *(Testimonies, Volume 9, 1909)*

496

The diet reform should be progressive. As disease in animals increases, the use of milk and eggs will become more and more unsafe. An effort should be made to supply their place with other things that are healthful and inexpensive. The people everywhere should be taught how to cook without milk and eggs so far as possible, and yet have their food wholesome and palatable.
(Ministry of Healing, 1905)

497

The science of cooking is not a small matter. The skillful preparation of food is one of the most essential arts. It should be regarded as among the most valuable of all the arts, because it is so closely connected with the life. Both physical and mental strength depend to a great degree upon the food we eat; therefore the one who prepares the food occupies an important and elevated position. *(Counsels to Teachers, 1913)*

"With guidance in meal planning, vegetarian diets are appropriate and healthful choices for adolescents. Vegetarian diets can also meet the needs of competitive athletes. Protein needs may be elevated because training increases amino acid metabolism, but vegetarian diets that meet energy needs and include good sources of protein (eg, soyfoods, legumes) can provide adequate protein without use of special foods or supplements. For adolescent athletes, special attention should be given to meeting energy, protein, and iron needs. Amenorrhea may be more common among vegetarian than nonvegetarian athletes, although not all research supports this finding."

Journal of the American Dietetic Association, November 1997, 97(1) citing the *American Journal of Clinical Nutrition,* 1991; 54:520–525, and *The Lancet,* 1984; 1:1474–1475.

498

Those who can avail themselves of the advantages of properly conducted, hygienic cooking schools, will find it a great benefit, both in their own practice and in teaching others. *(Christian Temperance and Bible Hygiene, 1890)*

499

Cooking schools are to be established in many places. This work may begin in a humble way, but as intelligent cooks do their best to enlighten others, the Lord will give them skill and understanding. The word of the Lord is, "Forbid them not; for I will reveal Myself to them as their Instructor." He will work with those who carry out His plans, teaching the people how to bring about a reformation in their diet by the preparation of healthful, inexpensive foods. Thus the poor will be encouraged to adopt the principles of health reform; they will be helped to become industrious and self-reliant. *(Testimonies, Volume 7, 1902)*

"Consuming fruit and vegetables was associated with a 27% lower stroke incidence, a 42% lower stroke mortality, a 24% lower ischemic heart disease mortality, a 27% lower cardiovascular disease mortality, and a 15% lower all-cause mortality. There is an inverse association of fruit and vegetable intake with the risk of cardiovascular disease and all-cause mortality in the general US population."

American Journal of Clinical Nutrition, 2002 Jul; 76(1):93–9

500

I have a well-set table on all occasions. I make no change for visitors, whether believers or unbelievers. I intend never to be surprised by an un-readiness to entertain at my table from one to half a dozen extra who may chance to come in. I have enough simple, healthful food ready to satisfy hunger and nourish the system. If any want more than this, they are at liberty to find it elsewhere. No butter or flesh meats of any kind come on my table. Cake is seldom found there. I generally have an ample supply of fruits, good bread, and vegetables. Our table is always well patronized, and all who partake of the food do well, and improve upon it. All sit down with no epicurean appetite, and eat with a relish the bounties supplied by our Creator.

(Testimonies, Volume 2, 1870)

Words to Live By . . .

I have written this to give you some idea of how we live. I never enjoyed better health than I do at the present time, and never did more writing. I rise at three in the morning, and do not sleep during the day. I would not use these health-destroying narcotics, for I prize health and I prize a healthful example in all these things. I want to be a pattern of temperance and of good works to others. My health is good. My appetite is excellent. I find that the simpler my food, and the fewer varieties I eat, the stronger I am. In our family we have breakfast at half past six o'clock, and dinner at half past one. We have no supper. We would change our times of eating a little, were it not for the fact that these are the most convenient hours for some of the members of the family. Our fare is simple and wholesome. We have on our table no butter, no meat, no cheese, no greasy mixtures of food. For some months a young man who was an unbeliever, and who had eaten meat all his life, boarded with us. We made no change in our diet on his account; and while he stayed with us he gained about twenty pounds. The food which we provided for him was far better for him than that to which he had been accustomed. All who sit at my table express themselves as being well satisfied with the food provided. *(1908 Letter)*

"Mrs. White has spoken on the health question in a manner to give entire satisfaction. Her remarks were clear and forcible, yet prudent, so that she carried the feelings of the entire congregation with her. On this subject, she always avoids extremes, and is careful to take only those positions where she is quite sure not to excite prejudices."

Review and Herald, November 8, 1870; Statement by Elder James White.

Concluding Thoughts

*N*ot long ago, my father, Nathan Cohen, suffered a stroke. Dad is a warrior who has always lived by that three-pronged sword otherwise known as a fork. Live by that sword, die by that sword. The Tuesday night before his stroke, Dad had been to a restaurant where he ordered the "steak-special"—a twenty-four-ounce New York cut that came from a cow and was finely marbled with delicious saturated animal fat. At the end of the meal, he splurged with some cheesecake for dessert.

During dinner, the acids in his stomach immediately went to work digesting that steak. After dinner, the cheesecake, with its high dairy content, neutralized the stomach acids, preventing proper digestion. Later that night, when indigestion and reflux threatened to rob him of a good night's sleep, my dad ate some ice cream—an old reliable self-treatment that always helped buffer the acid in his stomach. The contents of his stomach then emptied into his small intestine, where the remaining food, along with extra-large doses of saturated fat, was absorbed into his bloodstream. After years of eating meals like this, a thick coating of fat had built up along the inner walls of an artery in his neck. Eventually, the blood supply to his brain was cut off, resulting in a stroke. Thankfully, he survived.

After leaving the hospital around mid-December, Dad was able to recuperate in a nursing home. I visited him each day. With the holidays around the corner, I came across his "Merry Christmas" menu, which promised a meal of roast prime rib of beef au jus, broccoli spears with cheese sauce, baked potato with sour cream, and coconut custard pie. I kid you not! Before he had the stroke, my father would have eaten this food with relish. But no more! Instead I brought him a healthy holiday meal to replace the artery-clogging poison that was being served that day. After all, it was that kind of unhealthy food that had put him there in the first place.

Dad has since discovered Boca Burgers, Morningstar Farm's "sausages," and other nonmeat alternatives. Soy Delicious chocolate ice cream is now his favorite. His breakfasts include fresh melon and other fruits, and he enjoys brown rice and dishes like eggplant with vegan mozzarella cheese for lunch and dinner. He has also discovered the power of green, red, orange, and yellow fruits and vegetables. Now, whenever he goes out for dinner, he frequents places like Veggie Heaven in Teaneck, New Jersey, for some of the best veggie chicken and beef in the New York metropolitan area. He is learning to substitute his former unhealthy foods (including comfort foods), with healthier yet satisfying choices.

My dad will be celebrating his eighty-eighth birthday soon. Motivated by the desire to hold his grandchildren's children, he expects to live another decade or more. And I believe he can do it! Should he continue to eat a plant-based diet, the layer of fat within his arteries will disappear. His arterial walls will become stronger and regain their elasticity. He will begin to reverse his heart disease, and continue to be the miracle man that he has always been. As a vegan, he now shows compassion both to animals and to his own body. He eats "magic" foods that contain healthful bioflavonoids and isoflavones. His diet includes lots of fiber and whole foods that contain living enzymes. The antioxidants in fresh fruits and vegetables will help cure my dad from within. His example will teach and inspire millions of people to eat better while sparing the lives of billions of animals.

After researching and compiling Ellen G. White's inspired nutritional advice in this book, I'd like to conclude with the following ten quotes from her writings. I consider them the Ten Rules for better health care.

Ten Rules for Better Health Care

Rule I

"These people have lived improperly on rich food. They are suffering as a result of indulgence of appetite. A reform in their habits of eating and drinking is needed. But this reform cannot be made all at once. The change must be made gradually." (Quotation #258)

Rule II

"It is the duty of the physician to see that wholesome food is provided, and it should be prepared in a way that will not create disturbances in the human organism." (Quotation #252)

Rule III

"Physicians who use flesh meat and prescribe it for their patients, should not be employed in our institutions, because they fail decidedly in educating the patients to discard that which makes them sick. The physician who uses and prescribes meat does not reason from cause to effect, and instead of acting as a restorer, he leads the patient by his own example to indulge perverted appetite. The physicians employed in our institutions should be reformers in this respect and in every other. Many of the patients are suffering because of errors in diet. They need to be shown the better way. But how can a meat-eating physician do this? By his wrong habits he trammels his work and cripples his usefulness." (Quotation #260)

Rule IV

"When a physician sees a patient suffering from disease caused by improper eating and drinking or other wrong habits, yet neglects to tell him of this, he is doing his fellow being an injury. Those who understand the principles of life should be in earnest in striving to counteract the causes of disease." (Quotation #268)

Rule V

"An important part of the nurse's duty is the care of the patient's diet." (Quotation #255)

Rule VI

"The patients are to be provided with an abundance of wholesome, palatable food, prepared and served in so appetizing a way that they will have no temptation to desire flesh meat. The meals may be made the means of an education in health reform. Care is to be shown in regard to the combinations of food given to the patients." (Quotation #256)

Rule VII

"Let fruit be placed on the table in abundance." (Quotation #259)

Rule VIII

"We must remember that the habits and practices of a lifetime cannot be changed in a moment. With an intelligent cook, and an abundant supply of wholesome food, reforms can be brought about that will work well. But it may take time to bring them about." (Quotation #265)

Rule IX

"The food placed before them must necessarily be more varied in kind than would be necessary in a home family. Let the diet be such that a good impression will be made on the guests. This is a matter of great importance. The patronage of a sanitarium will be larger if a liberal supply of appetizing food is provided." (Quotation #264)

Rule X

"Fresh air, exercise, pure water, and clean, sweet premises, are within the reach of all, with but little expense; but drugs are expensive, both in the outlay of means, and the effect produced upon the system." (Quotation #273)

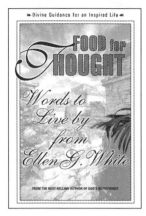

»– Divine Guidance for an Inspired Life –«

FOOD FOR THOUGHT

Words to Live By from Ellen G. White

Edited by Robert Cohen

As a spiritual leader, prolific writer, and pioneering nutritionist of the nineteenth and twentieth centuries, Ellen G. White had a profound effect on millions of people around the world. Today, her words continue to guide and inspire countless individuals. Although she is the most translated author in the history of American literature, few people outside the Seventh-day Adventist Church have known of her work—that is, until now. In this all-encompassing book, Robert Cohen presents Ellen White's most insightful thoughts on all aspects of life, from building strong character and recognizing the importance of family ties to dealing with disappointments and respecting the rights of animals.

Here then, are over 400 inspiring quotations from the writings of Ellen G. White that are as practical, insightful, and moral as they are accurate. Offering additional food for thought on her wide-ranging views are the words of other great luminaries from both the past and present. Paired with each of White's inspiring words of wisdom are the fascinating voices of such noteworthy individuals as William Shakespeare, Thomas Edison, Florence Nightingale, Mother Teresa, and Oprah Winfrey. Gathered from Mrs. White's many works, the classic quotations presented in this book are arranged topically and alphabetically in an easy-to-follow format.

Whether viewed as a unique slice of history, a book of prophetic wisdom, or a relevant guide to everyday life, *Food For Thought* offers both a beacon of light and a path of truth.

About the Author

Ellen G. White was a founder of the Seventh-day Adventist Church. Born in 1827, in Gorham, Missouri, her spiritual calling began at an early age. For the remainder of her life, she conducted a public ministry, traveling around the country and the world, spreading her revolutionary Christian thinking. In 1863, the Seventh-day Adventist Church was established and she became its first spiritual leader. Through her inspired guidance, what began as a handful of believers has grown to include millions of followers throughout the world.

$16.95 U.S./$25.50 CAN • 5.5-x-8.5-inch quality paperback •Religion/Lifestyle/Quotations • ISBN: 0-7570-0178-5